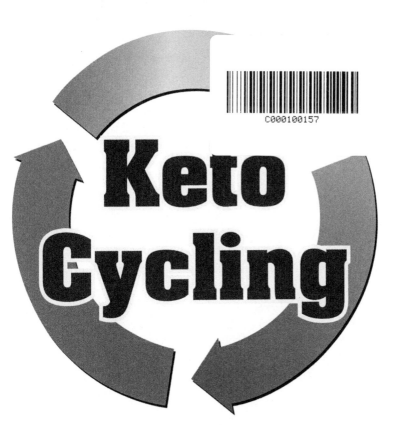

Keto Cycling

How To Optimize the Ketogenic Diet and Avoid Common Mistakes

Dr. Bruce Fife

P B

Piccadilly Books, Ltd.
Colorado Springs, CO

Every effort has been made to ensure that the information contained in this book is complete and accurate. However, neither the publisher nor the author is engaged in rendering professional advice or services to the individual reader. The information contained in this book is not intended as a substitute for consulting with your physician. All matters regarding your health require medical supervision. Neither the author nor the publisher shall be liable or responsible for any loss or damage allegedly arising from any information or suggestion in this book.

Piccadilly Books, Ltd.
P.O. Box 25203
Colorado Springs, CO 80936, USA
www.piccadillybooks.com
info@piccadillybooks.com

Library of Congress Cataloging-in-Publication Data

Names: Fife, Bruce, 1952 May 28- author.
Title: Keto cycling : how to optimize the ketogenic diet and avoid common mistakes / by Dr. Bruce Fife.
Description: Colorado Springs, CO : Piccadilly Books, Ltd., [2019] | Includes bibliographical references and index.
Identifiers: LCCN 2019020511 | ISBN 9781075462702
Subjects: LCSH: Ketogenic diet--Popular works. | Low-carbohydrate diet. | Self-care, Health--Popular works.
Classification: LCC RM237.73 .F54 2019 | DDC 641.5/6383--dc23
LC record available at https://lccn.loc.gov/2019020511

Printed in the USA

Table of Contents

Chapter 1: **Introduction** 5

Chapter 2: **The Miracle of Fasting** 12

Chapter 3: **The Ketogenic Diet** 26

Chapter 4: **Traditional Diets** 43

Chapter 5: **Keto Cycling** 63

Chapter 6: **The Healing Process** 87

Chapter 7: **Low-Calorie Sweeteners** 101

Chapter 8: **Keto Myths, Mistakes, and Misconceptions** ... 118

Chapter 9: **Fasting Mimicking Diet Recipes** 142

Appendix: **Keto Bookshelf** 150

References 168

Index 174

1

Introduction

In recent years, the ketogenic diet has gained a great deal of attention and for good reason. The diet has proven highly successful as a weight loss aid and as a means for reversing chronic degenerative disease. As good as the ketogenic diet is, its effects can be enhanced through the process of keto cycling: a method patterned after natural law in which a person alternates into and out of ketosis on a regular basis.

The ketogenic diet shifts the body into a natural, healthy metabolic state known as nutritional ketosis. In nutritional ketosis the body uses fat as its primary source of energy in place of glucose (sugar). Some of this fat is converted into ketones—high-potency fuel that boosts energy and cellular efficiency. When a person is in nutritional ketosis, special enzymes and genes that regulate cell survival and internal cleansing are activated or "switched on." When the body shifts back to burning glucose (glucosis), a different set of enzymes and genes that stimulate growth and healing are activated instead. Shifting between glucosis and ketosis continually activates these switches,upregulating or downregulating enzymes and genes stimulating healing and repair. As a consequence, blood pressure normalizes, blood cholesterol levels improve, excess weight and body fat melts off, energy levels increase, blood sugar and insulin levels normalize, memory and cognitive skills improve, and hormone levels improve. In short, the entire body feels the positive effects.

Keto cycling enhances the power of the ketogenic diet and makes it more user-friendly by allowing periods of time with higher carbohydrate intake and a greater variety of food choices. Many people feel the ketogenic diet is too restrictive, being very low in carbohydrate and high in fat with only moderate protein consumption. Keto cycling allows a more varied diet, with restrictions limited to only certain periods of time. Keto cycling spans a range from short or intermittent fasts to feasting on almost any type of food (though preferably still nutritious foods). The main goal is to move between glucosis and ketosis and back again, completing the cycle.

People are discovering that keto cycling is a powerful tool that can help them improve their health and better their lives.

"My story starts in 1993, where a routine medical test for life insurance discovered elevated protein levels in my urine," says Jerry. Elevated protein is a sign of possible kidney disease, which can be caused by elevated blood sugar levels or diabetes. "I was diabetic and needed to seriously reduce my blood glucose levels as my A1C reached a personal high of 7.4." A1C is a test that measures average blood glucose over a three month period. Levels between 4 and 5.6 are considered normal. Levels between 5.7 and 6.4 indicate prediabetes and levels of 6.5 or higher are a marker for diabetes.

Jerry began to follow the Diabetic Glycemic Diet to control his blood sugar levels. He used a glucose meter to read his sugar levels throughout the day. His blood sugar levels were erratic even with the diet. Medication was necessary to help bring them under control. Jerry went online to learn more about diabetes and diabetic medications. Here he learned about treating diabetes using a low-carb, high-fat diet. He felt he had nothing to lose by trying the diet along with periods of intermittent fasting—in essence, a form of keto cycling.

"My results were immediate," says Jerry. His blood glucose, as indicated by A1C test, dropped out of the diabetes zone into the 5 to 6 range. In just a few months his weight fell from 257 to 211 pounds (116 to 96 kg). He began the diet at the end of the year, but was able to adjust the fasting and eating cycles around Christmas, New Year's, birthdays, and special family dinners without feeling deprived or ostracized. The diet was flexible and easier than he had imagined.

At times, when he was eating and overdid it, his blood sugar levels would begin to inch up, but he wasn't concerned. He knew that a few days of fasting would quickly correct the problem. "I actually look forward to my fasting period," he says. It helps motivate him to stick with the program as he can see immediate results.

Lifestyle or dietary diseases, like type 2 diabetes, are not successfully treated with drugs. Drugs usually only treat the symptoms, not the disease itself. When the drugs fail to stop the disease, we are told the condition is chronic, there is no cure, and the only thing you can do is manage it with the use of drugs. In the meantime, the disease continues to progress. Keto cycling, on the other hand, offers a drugless solution that can produce far better results and, in some cases, even a cure.

At age 48, Kristy was diagnosed with type 2 diabetes. She was initially prescribed one medication for treatment, but over time she required more medications to control her blood sugar. By the age of 55, she was taking three medications for diabetes, as well as cholesterol-lowering, blood pressure, and heartburn medications—six medications in all.

Her brother, Scott, had struggled with type 2 diabetes for over 20 years, having been diagnosed when he was in his 30s. His diabetes was so severe that his pancreas could no longer function correctly, and he required insulin to control his blood sugar, injecting 70 units of insulin a day. At the age of 51, however, Scott was able to reverse his diabetes, getting completely off insulin and Metformin using a ketogenic diet and keto cycling.

Encouraged by her brother's successes, Kristy started the ketogenic diet along with fasting three separate days a week for 24 hours each. Her blood sugar levels responded immediately, dropping down within the prediabetic range. After just two weeks she no longer needed her diabetic medications and was able to discontinue all three of them. Her blood sugar levels were better with the diet than it had ever been when she was taking the medications. Other health issues also responded. Her weight and waist size decreased, heartburn disappeared, blood pressure normalized, and cholesterol values improved. After one month, she was able to discontinue all six of her medications. Kristy felt better than she had in years. She had no difficulty with the dietary protocol, including the periods of fasting. The ketogenic diet depressed her hunger and stifled food cravings to the point that fasting was not difficult or uncomfortable.

Keto cycling is useful for a wide variety of health problems, not just diabetes. "Several years ago, I was experiencing fatigue, especially after any physical exertion," recalls George. "My heart would pound rapidly and I felt lightheaded at times. In addition, I often had indigestion or would feel bloated. At 56, I thought maybe my age was catching up with me. I was diagnosed with cardiomyopathy—a form of heart disease that makes it harder for the heart to pump blood and can lead to heart failure. My blood sugar was also high, the doctor said I was prediabetic. I was put on drugs (ACE inhibitor and beta blocker) and told to eat a low-fat diet.

"I followed the doctor's instructions, watched what I ate, and started an exercise program—working out four days a week. After nearly two years there wasn't much improvement. I was still overweight, prediabetic, and my symptoms seemed worse.

"Looking for information about ways to reduce insulin resistance and improve heart health I learned about the low-carb, high-fat diet. After a year on the diet, I made some improvement, but still had a long way to go. I then found a website about intermittent fasting. When I combined that with my low-carb diet the improvement was dramatic.

"In a year and a half I've experienced the following benefits: much more energy, normal heartbeat (no more racing heart), loss of 55 pounds (25 kg) even though I reduced the amount of time I exercise, no more indigestion/bloating, reduced blood pressure, increased HDL (the good cholesterol), reduced blood triglycerides, reduced fasting blood sugar (no longer prediabetic), sleep better, and no longer need medications for my heart."

Most people start the ketogenic diet as a means to lose excess weight because it has proven to be far more effective than the standard low-fat, calorie-restricted diet. Brenda struggled with weight problems for most of her life, even as a child.

"I developed polycystic ovary syndrome (PCOS) and insulin resistance by my twenties with a diagnosis that I would surely become diabetic by 30," says Brenda. She followed her doctor's instructions and ate a low-fat, calorie-restricted diet and exercised daily. With a great deal of effort, she managed to achieve a normal weight, but could not get rid of her belly fat, even though there was little fat anywhere else.

Eventually, she gave up the struggle and decided to "eat normally" like everyone else, but with healthy, whole foods. Although she still worked out over an hour daily, she gained 75 pounds (34 kg) in eight months. She went to three endocrinologists and two nutritionists who all said she wasn't following the program correctly. When she insisted she was, they accused her of lying about how much she was eating and exercising. If she was doing everything right, she couldn't be gaining weight, she must be doing something wrong.

Brenda was put on Metformin and Byetta, which caused her to vomit daily. As a result, she lost 25 pounds (11 kg) but her blood sugar levels were still elevated. She couldn't stand the vomiting and after two years stopped taking the medication. She quickly regained the 25 pounds she had lost. Over the next few years and after the birth of two children, she gained another 46 pounds (21 kg) reaching a total of 256 pounds (116 kg).

The dietary advice from her physician wasn't helpful: it was the same old low-fat, calorie-restricted diet with regular exercise she had struggled with before. She decided to follow some of the current dietary fads by dropping gluten and dairy, but that didn't help. A friend of hers told her about the success people were having with the ketogenic diet. "I decided to try it," says Brenda. "I lost almost 40 pounds (18 kg) over 18 months, putting me at 217 (98 kg). I loved starting keto; I ate fats for the first time!"

Although she did well initially and lost weight, over time her progress stalled and her weight wouldn't budge. By this time, Brenda was diagnosed with full-blown diabetes with an A1C of 9, so she was put on insulin. She became pregnant again, but had a miscarriage.

A friend of hers described his positive experience with fasting as part of a church-sponsored retreat. This motivated her to give fasting a try. After fasting for a few days she lost 10 pounds (4.5 kg) and felt an increase in mental clarity. Over the next eight months she fasted multiple times, with her longest fast extending to eight days in a row, though she generally fasted three to four days per week. When she ate, she usually did keto or a single daily meal (intermittent fasting) going through a range of keto, fasting, and refeeding or keto cycling. Her A1C was retested and came in at 5.8—she was no longer diabetic. She slimmed down to 185 pounds (84 kg) on a 5'9" (175 cm) frame and continued to lose weight. More importantly, her belly fat that previously refused to budge was melting off.

Belly fat is known as visceral fat. This is the fat that is stored within the abdominal cavity, it is not the same as the fat that collects under your skin and hangs on around your thighs, butt, and arms. Instead, visceral fat accumulates around your organs—the liver, heart, and intestines. This causes the belly or waistline to bulge out. Visceral fat is not just excess fatty tissue, but metabolically active tissue that releases hormones, promotes inflammation, and increases the risk of a number of health problems, including obesity, heart disease, diabetes, cancer, depression, arthritis, hormonal imbalance, sleep disorders, and dementia. Waist circumference is a better predictor of cardiovascular disease and early death than is body weight. People who have a larger waist, whether they are overweight or not, are at a higher risk of health problems than those with a smaller waist. Through keto cycling, abdominal fat is effectively reduced, thus reducing the risk of a multitude of chronic health problems.

If done properly, the ketogenic diet is the most powerful, most effective, most efficient tool for overcoming chronic disease and restoring health. It is absolutely the easiest and most efficient method of losing excess body fat and eliminating belly fat.

Despite the proven effectiveness and general appeal of the ketogenic diet, there are people who have become discouraged with it. Too often I hear people lament, "Oh, I tried the keto diet but it didn't work for me." It didn't work? Why not? This diet has proven highly successful for countless numbers of people, has been demonstrated to be effective for weight loss and many other health issues through rigorous scientific research. Why do some people claim it doesn't work?

Most people who fail to see the results they expected from the diet were given faulty advice or had some misconceptions that affected the outcome. This is far more common than you might suspect.

There are a lot of myths and misinformation about the ketogenic diet on the Internet and even in books. Journalists often perpetuate these myths when they write about the diet in magazine articles. Many people seeing the growing popularity of the keto craze have jumped on the bandwagon and churned out recipe and weight loss books without really understanding what the diet is really all about. In fact, many of these recipes are not actually ketogenic. A common misconception is that the keto diet is simply a low-carb diet with a little more fat. However, typical low-carb recipes often contain too much protein, not enough fat, or too much carbohydrate to be effective for a keto diet. So, how much should or could you eat when doing keto? What types of foods should you eat, and which foods should you avoid? Which fats are best and which should be avoided? How can you tell when you are in ketosis? Do you even need to be in ketosis? How long should you stay on the diet? Should the diet be a lifelong change or should you end it after reaching your goal? What about keto cycling? What is it, and how can it benefit people on a ketogenic diet? These are very important questions and concerns that need to be answered in order to be successful with the ketogenic diet. Finding answers can be confusing because of conflicting information. The purpose of this book is to help you find the answers to these questions so that you can get the most benefit from the ketogenic diet and keto cycling.

2

The Miracle of Fasting

HISTORICAL PERSPECTIVE

Many people are skeptical of fasting. To them it is nothing more than starvation and unhealthy. We are told that we need three meals a day to be healthy and to keep up our strength. Missing a single meal makes you feel famished and weak and may cause a headache. It is unimaginable going an entire day without eating. Even many doctors discourage it.

Generally, it is believed that a person can only last five or six days without any food before becoming emaciated and die of starvation. However, while it is true that you cannot survive more than five or six days without water, the same is not true for food. As long as you have sufficient water to drink, you can survive without a single morsel of food for many weeks and even months. A normal weight person can survive for 6 to 8 weeks without any food if they are otherwise in good health and are adequately hydrated.

If we don't eat anything for awhile, our body relies on its storage of fat to supply its energy needs. That's why we lose weight on a calorie-restricted diet. The more body fat you have, the longer you can survive without food. It is not uncommon for medically supervised fasts, during which the patient consumes only water, to last 30 to 60 days. The longest supervised fast I am aware of is that of 26-year old Angus Barbieri, who fasted for over a year—382 days to be exact. His case was reported in a medical journal in 1973.[1]

At the beginning of the fast Barbieri weighed 456 pounds (207 kg). After consuming nothing but water and some vitamins and minerals for 382 days, he slimmed down to 180 pounds—a loss of 276 pounds. Barbieri was not laid up in bed, nor did he suffer any undue discomfort. Throughout the fast, he maintained his normal daily activities. In fact, the lack of food didn't even cause him agonizing hunger pangs or discomfort. Feelings of hunger generally fade after the first few days of a fast. "Apart from feeling a wee bit weak, I feel no ill effects," Barbieri reported at the end of his fast. The medical literature contains several case reports of fasts lasting 200 days or more.[2-4] All of which were done primarily for weight loss.

Some people claim that fasting is unnatural and will cause harm by making you weak and susceptible to disease. Fasting, however, is very natural. Our bodies are well adapted to going for periods of time with little or no food, storing up reserves of fat for anticipated lean periods. The primary purpose of body fat is to have a reserve of energy to sustain us during times when food is scarce or not available.

Throughout human history, obtaining food has been a struggle and there were many times when it was not available. Even when game was plentiful, a successful hunt was never guaranteed. Hunters would go out in search of game and take days to bring back enough meat for the family or community. In between these hunts, the community had to fast or rely on what was left over from previous hunts or whatever roots, grubs, and berries they could find in the meantime.

Between successful hunts, food was limited. The people would subsist in a semi-fasting state and if things got worse, as they often did in those days, they would have nothing at all to eat. When the hunt was successful, however, they would feast. These periods of feasting, semi-fasting, and complete fasting all varied in duration according to circumstances. This has been the normal order of things from the beginning of time. Even our more recent ancestors who planted crops and raised livestock could not guarantee a steady source of food, as they too suffered from food shortages during times of winter, famine, and drought. It has only been over the past 100 years or so that food has been steadily available for those with even a modest income. Today foods are prepared and packaged to have a long shelf life and shipped to and from all parts of the the world. Eating three meals a day, every day is a relatively recent development in human history. It is not fasting that is unnatural, eating three meals a day is unnatural! And it leads to ill health.

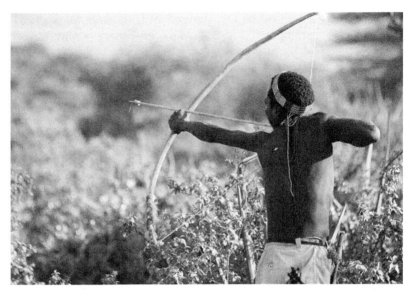

The hunt for food.

THERAPEUTIC FASTING

Fasting is a natural instinct. Animals intuitively fast whenever they are sick or injured. Even when food is available, they will refuse to eat until their health has improved. This is one way zoo caretakers indentify sick animals. By the same means, we know when our own pets are sick. Humans also have this instinct, but we often ignore it. Even though we may not feel hungry when sick, we are told we must eat something to "keep up our strength." So we load the body up with food, which requires energy to digest, energy that could better be used for healing the body.

Fasting is the oldest form of medicine. It was practiced by our primitive hunter-gatherer ancestors. They were more in tune with their instincts and knew from first-hand experience that fasting had a remarkable power to overcome illness and promote healing. The ancient Greek, Roman, and Egyptian philosophers and physicians advocated fasting as the primary tool or means to improve both mental and physical health. It was prescribed to cleanse the blood, sharpen the mind, and restore health to the sick.

Great religious leaders throughout history recognized the value of fasting in developing mental clarity and spiritual insight, and it remains a common practice in many religions. The ancient Romans used fasting as a means to dispel "demons" from people afflicted with delusions and hallucinations. These individuals (who likely suffered from epilepsy or schizophrenia) were locked in a room without food for several days. When their abnormal behavior ceased, it was an indication that the demons had left them. Although the Romans had no idea why locking afflicted people in a room caused the "evil spirits" to leave, in many cases, it worked.

Throughout history fasting has been used by physicians as a means to treat all forms of illness with varying degrees of success. Famed 16th century Swiss-German physician Paraceisus, claimed fasting to be the greatest remedy, calling it "the physician within us." The use of fasting therapy waxed and waned over the years as new medicines and procedures came into use. In the late 1800s and early 1900s, therapeutic fasting experienced a renewed surge in popularity, partly due to the ineffectiveness of the drugs used at the time and partly because it proved to be effective when other methods were not. Sanitariums, which treated chronic disease and relied on healthy foods and fasting as their major forms of treatment, sprang up all across America and Europe.

In 1920, if you had tuberculosis or cancer, you could go to a sanitarium and stay in a hospital-like setting attended by doctors and nurses. As part of your treatment, you would be exposed to fresh air, sunshine, healthy foods, and often fasting. The periods of fasting would vary from 3 to 40 days or even longer. Fasting was often repeated until the desired results were achieved. In a sanitarium of the period, fasting always included water and, in some cases, fresh fruit and vegetable juices as well. Moderate exercise was generally recommended during the fast and often involved a daily walk of anywhere from 2 to 10 miles or more.

Fasting therapy proved successful in treating a wide variety of health issues including digestive problems, arthritis, diabetes, prostate enlargement, liver disease, kidney disease, hormonal and reproductive problems, asthma, hypertension, epilepsy, cancer, psychological disorders, and much more. It is no wonder why fasting therapy became so popular. Studies published in more recent years have confirmed the effectiveness of fasting in treating a wide range of conditions.[5-11]

In the early 1900s many popular books were written advocating therapeutic fasting. One of the most outspoken proponents of fasting was American bodybuilder Bernarr Macfadden, the founder of the physical culture movement, which advocated exercise, natural foods, and drugless therapies for improved health and healing. He founded *Physical Culture* magazine in 1899 and wrote over 100 books on various aspects of health including *Fasting, Hydropathy, and Exercise* (1900) and *Fasting for Health* (1923).Born in 1868, Macfadden was a weak and sickly child and described himself as a "physical wreck." Through exercise, natural foods, and fasting he was able to turn his life around to become the poster boy of optimal health.

Another influential fasting advocate at the time was novelist Upton Sinclair. Sinclair suffered for years from chronic headaches, digestive distress, constipation, and numerous colds. He tried all types of diets and remedies without success. His diet was very restrictive because so many foods caused him problems. After learning about fasting therapy through the writings of Bernarr Macfadden and others, he went on several fasts from 10 to 12 days duration and found great relief. He was even able to reintroduce foods that had previously caused him trouble. "Bananas, acid fruits, peanut butter—I tried them one by one, and then in combination, and so realized with a thrill of exultation that every trace of my old trouble was gone," he said. "Formerly I had to lie down for an hour or two after meals; now I could do whatever I chose. Formerly I had been dependent upon all kinds of laxative preparations; now I forgot about them. I no longer had headaches. I went bareheaded in the rain, I sat in cold drafts of air, and was apparently immune to colds. And, above all, I had that marvelous, abounding energy so that whenever I had a spare minute or two I would begin to stand on my head, or to 'chin' myself, or do some other 'stunt,' from sheer exuberance of animal spirits." Sinclair described his experience in an article published in *Cosmopolitan* magazine. The article received such an overwhelming response that he was compelled to write a follow-up story. Soon after he wrote a book titled *The Fasting Cure* (1911), filled with over 270 success stories from others who had used fasting to overcome various health problems.

For example, one letter sent to Sinclair reads: "I wish to acknowledge my indebtedness to you for a restoration to such health of body and clarity of mind as I have not known since my sixteenth year, when first I entered the high school. That was twenty years ago...I quit eating on May 13 and did not take anything except water until the morning of May 26. Even then I was not hungry, but as I did not care to remain away from work any longer I broke the fast on the morning of the 26th. I lost thirteen pounds in weight, but was never too weak not to move around. I worked in the office for seven days, and the balance of the time remained at home, basking in the sunshine and reading constantly.

"As a result of the fast, I have sloughed off all my impedimenta of disease. Constipation of tens years' standing is gone as if by magic. Piles and resulting pruritis of eight years' tearing torture are nightmares of the past. Bronchitis and eczema of scalp have vanished. Asthma, due to nervous sympathy with the pneumogastric nerve (vagus nerve), is no more. Catarrhal deafness, sore throat, intestinal catarrh, and a general neurasthenic condition have left me. Work was never so pleasant. I cannot get enough of physical exercise, it seems; my muscles seem to grow stronger as the exercise proceeds...[I am] now in the full possession of physical health and mental strength which have come back to me."

Most of the other cases, many reporting fasts as long as 30 days, describe similar dramatic improvements in health.

With the eventual development of antibiotics, insulin, and other drugs, it was far easier for patients to take a pill or get a shot then it was to take time off work, check into a sanitarium, and go on a 30-day water fast, which might have to be repeated for full effect. Additionally, drug therapy proved far more profitable for the medical and pharmaceutical industries, and medical schools focused on drug treatments, generally ignoring fasting therapy. As a consequence, the vast majority of physicians today don't know much about fasting and often even advise against it.

Current medical research is now rekindling interest in therapeutic fasting. For instance, researchers at the Intermountain Medical Center Heart Institute in Salt Lake City have demonstrated that routine periodic fasting improves blood cholesterol and triglyceride levels, blood sugar, and body weight, and effectively reduces the risk of heart disease, diabetes, and obesity.[12]

The research team also discovered that in a test population of 200 individuals, a 24-hour water only fast increased the levels of human growth hormone (HGH) by an average of 1,300 percent in women and nearly 2,000 percent in men. This is remarkable and highly significant. HGH has a reputation of being an anti-aging hormone. The hormone is involved in building muscle and bone mass, sustaining healthy energy levels, and preventing excess fat accumulation. Many athletes and bodybuilders use HGH hormone injections to build muscle and enhance athletic performance. The hormone also supports healthy pancreatic, liver, and immune function; sharpens memory and cognitive abilities; reduces the risks of heart disease and diabetes; and aids in healing and tissue repair.

HGH is essential for the proper growth and development in children. As we age, levels decline. Consequently, with aging we tend to gain body fat, lose muscle and bone mass, have less energy, experience memory deficits, and become more susceptible to injury and infections. Some older adults, in an effort to reverse these trends and recapture some of the vitality and appearance of their youth, get medically supervised HGH injections. The hormone used for medical purposes is a synthetic version, is expensive, and is often accompanied by undesirable side effects. You can accomplish the same result naturally, without the side effects or expense, simply by fasting. It is no wonder why fasting therapy has been so highly regarded throughout the ages.

CALORIE RESTRICTION

Modified fasts, such as juice fasting (which includes both water and diluted fruit and vegetable juices) and very low-calorie diets (less than about 600 calories/day) have also proved to be very therapeutic with similar health benefits. In fact, most fasting clinics began using juice fasting in place of strict water fasting because it produced quicker results and provided enough energy for patients to be more active physically. The addition of vitamins, minerals, and a small amount of energy provided by the daily consumption of fresh juice boosted the body's cleansing and recuperative processes. For instance, water fasting was commonly used in the treatment of cancer. Although this approach was effective in stopping or slowing the growth of the cancer, it didn't always get rid of it. Adding fresh juices provided the body with the nutrients and the energy that it needed to more effectively fight off the cancer, resulting in an increased success rate. This led to experiments with underfeeding or calorie restriction.

In animals, studies have shown that underfeeding as opposed to overeating tends to delay age-related diseases and prolong life. Studies as far back as 1915 reported that restricting the food intake of rodents resulted in a considerable increase in their lifespan. This observation was explored in more detail in the 1930s by C.M. McCay and colleagues at Cornell University. McCay learned that underfed rodents were generally healthier and lived up to 40 percent longer than their well-fed counterparts. In certain species of worms, the results are even more dramatic. When given continual access to abundant food, the worms pass through their whole life in three to four weeks, but when the food was greatly reduced or they were forced to fast periodically, they would continue to be active and young for over three years. The additional years of life aren't just an extension of old age but rather are an extension of their youth. For example, mice that were the equivalent of 90 years of age in terms of human years could still be fertile and produce young. Over the years, calorie restriction has been shown to significantly extend the healthy life of fruit flies, worms, mice, fish, monkeys, and other animals.

Calorie restriction is often referred to as an "anti-aging diet" because it slows the aging process and extends lifespan. It also provides protection against numerous degenerative diseases that tend to shorten life. For example, one published report showed that breast cancer incidence fell from 40 percent in fully fed animals to only 2 percent in calorie-restricted animals; lung cancer fell from 60 to 30 percent; liver cancer fell from 64 to 0 percent; and cardiovascular disease fell from 63 to 17 percent.[13]

Other conditions that are delayed or avoided by calorie restriction include arthritis, diabetes, atherosclerosis, Alzheimer's, and virtually all age-related degenerative diseases.[14-15]

In animal studies, 40 to 50 percent calorie restriction has produced the greatest extension in lifespan. In humans, restricting calories this much is too difficult to maintain. A 25 percent restriction is more double; a normal 2,000-calorie diet would be reduced to 1,500 calories. Even still, it takes a great deal of willpower to maintain this level of restriction for life. At this level, human studies have reported improvement in various measures of health status, similar to those seen in animal studies. A change in maximum lifespan has not yet been determined because the studies have not gone on long enough.

Since the total amount of food is decreased, what is eaten must be nutrient dense, and empty calories like those found in most commercially processed foods must be avoided. Eating empty calories on a restricted diet will lead to malnutrition. This is why semi-starved populations in certain parts of world don't live longer—they are both calorie-restricted and malnourished.

There are some people who have followed a calorie-restricted diet continually for over 20 years. While this is far too short of a time to determine what effect it has on human longevity, what has been shown is that many of the markers doctors measure to evaluate a patient's health improve over this time. For example, blood pressure is normalized, blood sugar and insulin levels decline and stabilize, systemic inflammation declines (as measured by C-reactive protein levels), body mass index improves, and heart rate slows down, all of which indicate a reduction in risk of common health problems such as diabetes and heart disease. While encouraging, not all of the changes have been positive. The habitual restriction of calories has led to some adverse effects such as infertility, chronic low energy, lowered immune response, and slowed healing of injuries. These symptoms are only temporary, as increasing calorie intake can reverse them.

One of the mistakes the early experimenters made was to eliminate fat from their diet. Fat contains more than twice as many calories as carbohydrate or protein, so to reduce total calorie intake as much as possible and yet allow for the greatest bulk of food, fat was almost completely eliminated. It was assumed that vegetables and grains contained all of the fat needed to avoid essential fatty acid deficiency. Consequently, fat intake was limited to only about 10 percent of total calories. Fat is a far more important nutrient then they realized and the lack of fat leads to hormonal imbalances and neurological and psychological disorders.

The most well-known advocate for calorie restriction was Roy L. Walford, MD, a professor of medicine at UCLA medical school. Based on animal research, Walford believed human lifespan could be extended to 120 years on a calorie-restricted diet. He wrote several best-selling books on the topic, including *The 120 Year Diet (1986)*and *The Anti-Aging Plan (1994)*. His plan was based on the concept of "calorie restriction with optimal nutrition" or what he termed "CRON." He claimed it would "retard the basic rate of aging in humans, greatly extending the period of youth and middle age, postpone the onset of such late-life disease as heart disease, diabetes, and cancer; and even lower the overall susceptibility to disease at any age."

In insects and animals eating their normal, but calorie-restricted diet, this appeared to be true. But in humans, the prejudice against fat led to deficiencies that seriously affected hormone levels and brain health. Walford began eating exclusively a low-fat, calorie-restricted diet when he was in his early 60s. He fully expected to live to be at least 100. However, after about 10 years he developed ALS, a brain wasting disease, and died at the age of 79.

Although adding more fat into a calorie-restricted diet may help prevent the hormonal changes and neurological deficits experienced by early calorie restriction practitioners, it might not completely prevent other symptoms such as a lack of energy, irregular or loss of menses and slow wound healing. The occurrence of these symptoms provides a clue that long term calorie restriction is not an optimal means of preserving health. Nor is it natural for humans to be in a continual state of calorie deficiency. Even our ancient ancestors who struggled to obtain food from day to day went through periods of *both* feasting and fasting.

Another important lesson learned from calorie restriction experiments is that having constant access to food leads to overfeeding, weight gain, and an increased risk of developing degenerative disease. Eating three meals a day, as we typically do, promotes obesity and ill health, which may help explain why chronic, degenerative disease is far more common today than it was in the past (see Chapter 4). Restricting calorie intake prevents this. But constant calorie restriction, especially if the diet is not optimal, can create problems too. A more natural, and healthful approach is to cycle through periods of feasting and fasting just as our ancestors did as part of their everyday existence.

THE ULTIMATE CLEANSER

The reduction in calorie consumption during a fast puts the body into a mild state of stress that triggers multiple survival mechanisms that flush out toxins and diseased tissue, reduce free-radical generation, calm inflammation, and slow aging. Fasting and periodic calorie-restricted dieting have shown to promote improved health and prevent degenerative changes that lead to chronic disease, which can improve the quality of life and potentially increase healthy lifespan.

We are constantly exposed to harmful microorganisms, environmental toxins, damaging chemicals, and pollutants. In addition, the cells in our bodies gradually age, accumulate debris, become dysfunctional, and die. A diet loaded with excessive calories, chemical additives and contaminants, and lacking in essential nutrients further burdens the body, leading to the accumulation of waste and the development of chronic disease.

Fasting is viewed as the ultimate cleanser. When the body isn't burdened with digesting and processing food, it is able to channel its energies to housecleaning and detoxification, and purging toxins. Our digestive system uses a great deal of energy; although it comprises less than 6 percent of the body's weight, it consumes up to 35 percent of our energy. In addition, the vast majority of the immune system is concentrated around the digestive tract to protect us from microbes that often find their way into our bloodstream. The immune system is always on alert around the digestive tract to battle incoming microorganisms. When we do not eat, most of this energy can be diverted to cleansing and healing throughout the body and remarkable things happen.

One of those things is the removal and replacement of old cells and tissues with new healthy stem cell-generated tissues. This process is called autophagy. Autophagy is essentially a form of self-cannibalism. As we go without food, tissues are called upon in the reverse order of their importance to the survival of the body to supply our ongoing energy needs. Fat, which is stored specifically for this purpose, is the first tissue to be used. As the body consumes its fat reserves, it then begins to dismantle old, dysfunctional, diseased, and damaged tissues and cells. In this process, useless and potentially harmful tissue, such as cancerous cells and tumors, are removed. As these become depleted, the skeletal muscles are the next to be tapped. Organs such as the brain, heart, and lungs, which are vital to life, are the last to be affected. In fact, even when death is caused by starvation, these vital organs retain all their functional ability and strength until the end.

One of the characteristics of Alzheimer's disease is the formation of sticky amyloid plague that collects in the brain. This plaque is believed to interfere with normal brain function and contribute to the symptoms associated with the disease. When fasting, this plaque is dissolved and removed, clearing the brain of this debris. The same occurs to plaque in the arteries and elsewhere throughout the body, reducing hypertension, atherosclerosis, and the risk of cardiovascular disease. Damaged cells, scar tissue, skin tags, and any cells that no longer serve a useful purpose are removed, recycled, and converted into glucose to supply the energy needed to keep more essential tissues functioning.

During the fast the body is in a state of intense housecleaning in which tissues are torn down and discarded or recycled. Tissue repair and growth actually slows down during this time. When the fast is over, the increased availability of energy (from glucose) and building materials (from fat and protein) shifts the body into a state of rebuilding. At this time, cleansing slows to a crawl and a period of growth and repair dominates. Old or damaged cells that were removed during the fast are replaced by new functional cells. As a result, many chronic health problems are resolved or greatly improved.

22

Fasting is much like renovating an old, rundown house. At first (the fasting phase), you go in to clean up the trash; scrub off dirt and stains from the floor and walls; scrape off peeling paint; remove rotted wood, broken tiles, and chipped bricks; and generally remove everything that is broken or worn out. Afterwards (the refeeding phase), you replace the damaged material with new wood, titles, and brick, fill in the cracks, and add a coat of paint and varnish. The building's former beauty and function is restored.

Long-term fasting or calorie restriction is not good because it doesn't allow for a period of rebuilding and healing to take place. Calorie restriction is like being in a continual state of housecleaning or tearing down and removal without the accompanying period of rebuilding, growth, and healing. Refeeding must follow every fast to complete the cycle.

When doing a water or juice fast it is customary to repeat the fast multiple times for maximum effect rather than do a single very long fast. Many people do fast for 30 or more days and experience remarkable results. Typically, even extended fasts often need to be repeated to get the desired results. It is usually easier to do multiple mid-length (7-14 days) or short (1-6 days) fasts. This way you go through the complete cleansing-rebuilding cycle multiple times. That said, some health problems do need longer fasts to completely remove diseased tissue. A mixture of short and longer fasts seems to work best.

INTERMITTENT FASTING

Water and juice fasting have proven to be extremely beneficial for losing weight and improving overall health; however, compliance can be difficult. As the first meal or two is missed, the stomach begins to groan and growl, pangs of hunger make themselves clearly known, and visions of tempting foods dance in your head. Your willpower is sorely tested. You want the health benefits that fasting can provide, but going without eating can be a struggle, especially initially as the body transitions from burning glucose to fat as its main source of fuel.

For this reason, intermittent fasting was developed to ease the discomfort of fasting but still provide many of the same benefits. Intermittent fasting is a general term used to describe a number of techniques that involve cycling in and out of fasting or semi-fasting over specified periods of time generally lasting from 16 to 24 hours. Since the duration of the fast is limited and separated by periods of normal eating, it is much easier for most people to follow. To make it effective, intermittent fasting needs to continue for a period of several months.

The most well-known intermittent fasting methods are:

• **Alternate-Day Fast**: Fast for 1 day and eat a normal diet the next. The fast day would be restricted to water only or consist of a modified fast of a single meal containing 600 or fewer calories. The single meal would generally be consumed at dinner time.

• **The 5:2 Diet**: Eat a normal diet for 5 days and fast for 2 (nonconsecutive) days per week. The fast day can be water only or consist of a modified fast of a single meal containing 600 or fewer calories.

• **Daily Time-Restricted Diet**: Food is consumed only during a 4 to 8 hour period of time each day. Nothing is consumed during the fast except water. The 16/8 method is the most popular. Here you fast for 16 hours straight and then are allowed to eat whatever you want for 8 hours. For example, if you finish eating dinner at 7:00 pm, you refrain from eating anything afterwards until 11:00 am the next morning—a fasting period of 16 hours. You can eat as much as you like between 11:00 am to 7:00 pm, when you start the cycle over again. A more intense version would increase the fasting period to 20 hours and restrict the eating time to just 4 hours a day.

There are many variations to these fasting methods. For example, the 5:2 diet could be modified to a 4:3 or a 6:1 diet. The daily time-restricted diet could increase the fasting time to 23 hours, allowing only 1 hour for a single meal each day. They have all shown to be beneficial for weight loss and improving health markers.

For short duration fasts of less than 1 or 2 days, as described above, water only is preferred over the modified fast as it produces better results. In fact, the longer the period of time without food, the better the results.

The primary goal of intermittent fasting is to reduce total calorie intake. Studies have shown that even though calorie consumption is only restricted during certain periods of time, this is enough to produce positive changes in body mass and metabolic health.

One might question that if you don't eat anything one day, the next day you will be so famished that you will overeat to make up for the missed meals. However, this doesn't happen. After a full day fast people don't eat any more than about 10 percent over what they would normally eat. Therefore, their total calorie intake is still about 45 percent less over the two days. The same is true when you limit your eating to just a few hours every day. When you do eat, you won't overeat to the extent that you make up for the calories you would have eaten in the missed meals.

It takes about 12 hours for the body to burn most of the sugar (glucose) stored in the liver as glycogen. Most people eat three meals a day and often snack in between. Therefore, they never deplete their glycogen stores. This conditions the body to use only sugar as fuel and effectively prevents the body from developing the ability to effectively use fat as fuel.

In order for intermittent fasting to work, the duration of the fast must be at least 12 hours long. The longer the better, as this is when the body is removing fat and cleansing. One drawback to intermittent fasting is that the limited period of time spent fasting does not allow significant time to thoroughly cleanse the body of waste and toxins to the extent that a water or juice fast does. It is great for weight loss and modest improvement in some health markers, but to reverse chronic health problems require longer fasts or the aid of a ketogenic diet, as described in Chapter 3.

Studies have shown that people lose weight and see a general improvement in health even when on "feast" days they eat their normal diet without regard to making healthy choices. Keep in mind that this is probably the type of food that caused the weight gain and poor health to begin with, so this is not the optimal choice. Limiting your calorie intake—regardless of the exact foods you do eat—will result in weight loss, but weight loss alone will not fix health problems. A healthy diet is also necessary and will greatly enhance the effects of the fast. Unfortunately, many people do not really understand what constitutes a truly healthy diet. The typical low-fat diet is not healthy. Healthy fats are essential for achieving good health. A high-carbohydrate diet is not particularly healthy either—it depends on the types of carbohydrate you eat as well as how the foods are processed and prepared. This topic is covered in the next chapter.

3

The Ketogenic Diet

THE CLASSIC KETOGENIC DIET

During the early 20th century, fasting therapy was used to treat a wide variety of difficult-to-treat health problems, one of which was epilepsy. Putting patients on a water-only fast for 10 to 30 days produced remarkable effects, resulting in a significant decrease in the intensity and the number of seizures they experienced. The positive results were not limited to just the period of time they were doing the fast, but lasted many months and even years afterword. Some even became seizure-free for the remainder of their lives, effectively curing the disorder completely—a rather remarkable achievement for a condition that was otherwise considered incurable.

One of the most outspoken proponents of fasting therapy for the treatment of epilepsy was Dr. Hugh Conklin, a Wisconsin osteopath. He recommended fasting for 18 to 25 days. He treated hundreds of epilepsy patients with his "water diet" and boasted a 90 percent cure rate in children and a 50 percent cure rate in adults.

Dr. H. Rawle Geylin, a prominent New York pediatrician, witnessed Conklin's success firsthand and tested the therapy on 36 of his own patients, achieving similar results. His patients ranged in age from 3.5 to 35 years. After fasting for 20 days, 87 percent of the patients were free of seizures. Geylin presented his findings at the annual meeting of the American Medical Association in Boston in 1921, ushering in fasting therapy as a mainstream treatment for epilepsy. In the 1920s when only phenobarbital and bromides were available as anticonvulsant medications, reports that fasting could cure epilepsy were exciting. These reports instigated a flurry of clinical investigations and research on fasting and epilepsy.

As a result of fasting therapy, many epileptic patients would remain seizure-free for years, if not for life. For others the cure was only temporary. In children, long-term freedom from seizures occurred in about 18 percent of cases. Repeating the fast would stop the seizures again, but there was no guarantee for how long. Longer fasts seemed to produce better results, but for some patients the length of time required to bring a lasting cure seemed impractical. Researchers began looking at ways to mimic the metabolic and therapeutic effects of fasting while allowing the patient to consume enough nourishment to sustain life and maintain good health for extended periods of time, and hopefully bring about a higher cure rate. The result of this research led to the development of the ketogenic diet.

The ketogenic diet severely restricted carbohydrate consumption, with a moderate restriction on protein as well. To maintain normal total calorie intake, the missing carbohydrate and protein were replaced with additional fat. The ketogenic diet can be summarized as one that is very low in carbohydrate, high in fat, with adequate protein to meet daily nutritional needs.

The ketogenic diet provided enough energy to support normal daily activities, even those requiring strenuous physical labor, as well as a full spectrum of essential nutrients to sustain normal growth (in adolescence) and healing. With the ketogenic diet, patients could remain in a metabolic state that was nearly equivalent to fasting for an indefinite period of time. Patients could stay on the diet for months and even years, if necessary, without suffering any long-term detrimental effects. Over the years the ketogenic diet proved highly successful in treating epilepsy, eliminating or greatly reducing seizure frequency and intensity for life even among those with very serious drug-resistant forms of the disease. Today, epileptic children undergoing ketogenic therapy are typically put on the diet for about 2 years before transitioning back to a normal diet.

Under normal conditions, our bodies burn glucose (sugar) for energy. We get glucose primarily from eating carbohydrates (starch and sugar), which are found abundantly in breads, grains, legumes, fruit, and some vegetables. During a fast (or a very low-calorie diet) when little or no food containing carbohydrate is consumed, body fat is taken out of storage and utilized to supply the body's continuous need for energy. This is why we lose weight during a fast or when dieting. During a fast, the body is powered by burning fat. The same is true for a ketogenic diet. Carbohydrate and protein are replaced by fat, shifting the body into a state of burning fat, thereby effectively mimicking the metabolic state of fasting without the severe calorie restrictions.

Some of this fat is converted by the liver into water-soluble compounds (beta-hydroxybutyrate, acetoacetate, and acetone), collectively known as "ketone bodies" or simply ketones. Normally, the brain uses glucose to satisfy its energy needs. Fats released from storage cannot pass over the blood-brain barrier to feed the brain; if glucose is not available, one of the only other sources of fuel the brain can use is ketones. Other organs and tissues in the body can utilize fat for energy, but not the brain—it must have either glucose or ketones. Ketones actually provide a more concentrated and efficient source of energy than glucose and have been described as our body's "superfuel," producing energy more efficiently than either glucose or fat.[1] It is like putting high-performance gasoline into the tank of your car—the engine runs more smoothly and cleanly, with better fuel efficiency. Ketones have a similar effect on the brain and other organs in the body.

Ketones also activate special proteins in the brain called brain derived neurotrophic factors (BDNF). These proteins regulate brain cell function, repair, and growth as well as calm inflammation and promote healing. As a consequence, the dysfunction or short circuit caused by epilepsy is overridden, and over time the brain is allowed to gradually rewire and heal itself.

The classic ketogenic diet developed in the 1920s contains a 4:1 ratio (3:1 for infants and teens) by weight of fat to combined protein and carbohydrate. This means each meal contains four times as much fat as it does a combination of both protein and carbohydrate. There are 9 calories in 1 gram of fat and 4 calories each in 1 gram of protein and 1 gram of carbohydrate. An unrestricted, ordinary diet consists of about 30 percent fat, 15 percent protein, and 55 percent carbohydrate. The 4:1 weight ratio of the ketogenic diet equates to about 90 percent of calories from fat, 8 percent from protein, and 2 percent from carbohydrate. As such, the ketogenic diet is a very high-fat program.

Carbohydrate consumption is restricted to 10 to15 grams per day. The diet excludes most high-carbohydrate grains, fruits, and vegetables, such as breads, corn, bananas, peas, and potatoes. Total calorie consumption is reduced to 80 to 90 percent of estimated energy requirements because this was believed to improve ketone levels. This hasn't been too much of a problem because ketones tend to reduce hunger so patients feel satisfied without feeling hungry.

Initially, fluid consumption was restricted to 80 percent of normal daily needs. This was done in the belief that it increased blood levels of ketones. However, the lack of fluid resulted in an increased risk of developing kidney stones. Later it was found that restricting fluid intake had no benefit and the practice was discontinued.

Since every calorie of fat, protein, and carbohydrate is precisely calculated and measured, the patient is required to eat the entire meal without receiving any extra portions. Every meal needs to have the 4:1 ratio. Any snacks have to be incorporated into the daily total calorie allotment and must have the same ratio. Consequently, it takes a good deal of time and effort to prepare meals and snacks.

Dr. Russel Wilder of the Mayo Clinic coined the term "ketogenic diet" to describe a diet that produced a high level of ketones in the blood through the consumption of a high-fat, low-carbohydrate diet. He was the first to use the ketogenic diet as a treatment for epilepsy.

Wilder's colleague, Mynie Peterman, MD, later formulated the classic 4:1 ketogenic diet. Peterman documented positive effects of improved alertness, behavior, and sleep with the diet in addition to seizure control. The diet proved to be very successful, especially with children. Peterman reported in 1925 that 95 percent of patients he studied had improved seizure control on the diet and 60 percent became completely seizure-free.

The ketogenic diet proved to be highly successful in treating epilepsy, including the most difficult drug-resistant forms. Over time, researchers began to wonder if the ketogenic diet could also be useful for other neurological disorders, so they tried it on patients with Alzheimer's disease, Parkinson's disease, multiple sclerosis (MS), ALS, traumatic brain injury, and stroke. In every case, the ketogenic diet proved highly effective. It was later discovered that the ketogenic diet was also beneficial in treating a wide variety of health problems including obesity, diabetes, heart disease, cancer, allergies, arthritis, digestive problems, and essentially all the diseases that fasting had been used for. After all, the diet was designed specifically to mimic the metabolic effects of fasting so it only makes sense that it would have many of the same therapeutic effects as well.

SUGAR METABOLISM
Carbohydrate is Sugar

We derive energy from the three major nutrients in our foods—carbohydrate, protein, and fat. While protein and fat can be used to produce energy, their primary function is to provide the basic building blocks for tissues, hormones, enzymes, and other structures that make up the human body. The primary purpose of carbohydrate, on the other hand, is to produce energy.

Carbohydrate is found in virtually all plant foods. Milk is the only animal-derived food that contains any appreciable carbohydrate. Plants are made predominantly of carbohydrate. The carbohydrate in our diet consist of some combination of three sugar molecules—glucose, fructose, and galactose. Table sugar or sucrose consists of one molecule of glucose and one of fructose. Lactose, or milk sugar, consists of one molecule of glucose and one of galactose. Starch, a major component of grains and certain vegetables such as potatoes and legumes, consists of long chains of glucose. Glucose is by far the most abundant sugar molecule in plant foods.

When food containing carbohydrate is consumed, digestive enzymes break the bonds between the sugar molecules, releasing the individual glucose, fructose, and galactose molecules. These sugars are then transported to the bloodstream. Here, glucose, also referred to as blood sugar, is delivered throughout the body to supply the fuel needed by the cells. Fructose and galactose in their current form cannot be used by the cells to produce energy. They are taken up by the liver, converted into glucose, and then released back into the bloodstream. Foods high in glucose produce a rapid rise in blood sugar concentration. Fructose and galactose increase blood sugar as well, but not as rapidly because they must pass through the liver first.

Most cells cannot store glucose. They take up and use only what is necessary for their immediate needs. The liver and muscle cells are exceptions; they have the ability to store a small amount of glucose in the form of glycogen for later use. The liver holds enough glycogen to supply our energy needs for about 12 hours, as glycogen levels drop the body begins to use fat to produce energy. Some of this fat is converted into ketones, primarily to fuel the brain, although the heart, skeletal muscles, and other organs can use them as well.

The Hormone Insulin

As glucose circulates throughout the body, it is picked up by the cells and converted into energy. The cells, however, cannot absorb glucose by themselves. They need the help of the hormone insulin. Insulin unlocks the door on the cell membrane which makes it possible for glucose to enter. Without insulin, glucose cannot enter the cells. Your blood could be saturated with glucose, but if insulin was not present, glucose could not pass though the cell membrane, and the cells would "starve" and die.

Every cell in your body needs a continuous supply of glucose to function normally. However, an overabundance of glucose is not good either. Too much glucose is toxic. In order to avoid the dire consequences of too little or too much glucose, the body has built in feedback mechanisms that maintain a narrow range of glucose levels in the blood.

Every time we eat, blood sugar levels rise. As sugar levels increase, special cells in the pancreas are triggered to release insulin into the bloodstream. As insulin shuttles glucose into the cells, blood sugar levels drop. At some point, another signal triggers the pancreas to stop insulin secretion. If blood sugar levels fall too low, the pancreas is prodded to release another hormone called glucagon. Glucagon induces the release of glucose stored in the liver, thus increasing blood sugar levels. In this way, blood sugar is continually maintained within a narrow boundary.

Blood sugar levels naturally fluctuate slightly throughout the day. Whenever we eat, blood sugar levels increase. Between meals or during times of heavy physical activity, as the body's demand for energy increases, blood sugar levels decline. As long as the body is capable of compensating for both upward and downward spikes in blood sugar, balance is maintained.

What we eat profoundly affects the workings of this system. High carbohydrate meals, especially if they contain a significant amount of sugar and a lack of fiber, fat, and protein, can cause blood glucose levels to rise very rapidly. Refined starches such as white flour, which have been stripped of most of their fiber and bran, tend to act like sugar, spiking blood glucose levels as well. The larger the quantity of simple and refined starch in meals, the greater the spike in blood sugar and the greater the strain placed on the body and especially the pancreas, which produces both opposing hormones—insulin and glucagon. Fiber, protein, and especially fat slow down the digestion and absorption of carbohydrate so glucose trickles gradually into the bloodstream, providing a steady, ongoing supply.

If a high carbohydrate meal is eaten every four or five hours, along with one or two high carbohydrate snacks such as a candy bar, soda, donut, or coffee with sugar between meals, insulin levels are going to be raised continually for a substantial part of the day. When cells are continually exposed to high insulin levels, they begin to lose their sensitivity to the hormone. It is like walking into a room with a bad odor. When you first enter the room the smell can be overpowering, but if you have to stay in the room for any length of time, the smell receptors in your nose become desensitized and you will not notice the odor any longer. The smell is still there, but your ability to detect the smell has declined. If you left the room for a while and your sense of smell became re-sensitized, as soon as you walked back into the room you would again notice the odor. Our bodies react in somewhat the same way with insulin. Chronic exposure to high insulin levels desensitizes the cells, and they become unresponsive or resistant to the action of insulin. This is referred to as *insulin resistance*. In an individual with insulin resistance, a higher than normal concentration of insulin is needed to move glucose into the cells, which puts more stress on the pancreas to produce more of the hormone. Insulin resistance is the first step toward developing diabetes. It is also the first step toward heart disease, Alzheimer's disease, and many other chronic degenerative diseases, including cancer. Diet, therefore, has a direct effect on the development of insulin resistance and consequently, on overall health.

Insulin Resistance and Diabetes

If you are an average, non-diabetic individual, when you wake up in the morning, your blood contains between 65 and 100 mg/dl (3.6-5.5 mmol/l) of glucose. This is known as the fasting blood glucose concentration. Fasting blood sugar measurements are taken after a person has not eaten for at least 12 hours. The ideal fasting blood sugar range is between 65-90 mg/dl (3.6-5.0 mmol/l).

When you don't eat and as your cells continue to draw glucose out of the blood, your glucose level gradually falls. Most people experience a feeling of hunger at about 65 mg/dl (3.6 mmol/l), the low end of the normal range. The normal response to this sensation is to eat, which raises blood sugar. Normally, your blood sugar should not rise to more than 139 mg/dl (7.7 mmol/l) after eating a meal. This is called postprandial glucose level. Elevated fasting and postprandial glucose levels indicate insulin resistance.

Diabetes is diagnosed when fasting blood sugar reaches 126 mg/dl (7.0 mmol/l) or higher. People with fasting blood sugar levels between 101 and 125 mg/dl (5.6-6.9 mmol/l) are considered to be in the early stages of diabetes, often referred to as "prediabetes." Fasting blood sugar levels over 90 mg/dl (5.0 mmol/l) indicate the beginning stages of insulin resistance. As insulin resistance increases, so do blood sugar levels. The higher the blood sugar, the greater the insulin resistance.

Insulin resistance is usually present in anyone who has a fasting blood sugar level over 90 mg/dl (5.0 mmol/l). Although levels up to 100 mg/dl (5.5 mmol/l) are generally considered to be "normal," they are viewed this way only because so many people fit into this category. Although blood sugar at this level is typical, it is not healthy. Having insulin resistance is not a state of health, even if the condition is relatively mild.

Over the past several decades, a tenfold increase in the incidence of type 2 diabetes has occurred worldwide. This is believed to be caused by the increased consumption of refined carbohydrates. Animal studies have shown that diets very high in sugar cause insulin resistance and diabetes. It is evident that the change in dietary habits in humans is at the core of our current diabetes epidemic.

Insulin Resistance and Brain Health

Insulin resistance can have an adverse effect on virtually every organ and system in the body. Nerves are particularly sensitive to elevated blood sugar and insulin levels. Chronic insulin resistance causes nerve damage leading to a condition known as diabetic neuropathy. Diabetic neuropathy is the most common serious complication of diabetes. About 60 to 70 percent of people with diabetes have some form of it. Symptoms include pain, tingling, or numbness in the hands, arms, feet, and legs. The legs and feet are most commonly affected, but nerve damage can develop throughout the body, including the brain.

Population-based studies have also shown that those with type 2 diabetes have an increased risk of cognitive impairment, dementia, and neurodegeneration.[2] The damage done to the nerves by insulin resistance increases the risk of developing Alzheimer's disease as well as other neurodegenerative diseases. Diabetics have almost twice the risk of getting Alzheimer's disease as the general population.[3] The younger a person is when he or she develops insulin resistance, the greater the risk. If diabetes occurs before the age of 65, it is associated with a 125 percent increased risk of eventually developing Alzheimer's disease.[4] Even pre-diabetics are in danger of developing Alzheimer's. The common denominator between pre-diabetes, diabetes, and Alzheimer's disease is insulin resistance.

The underlying cause of type 2 diabetes—insulin resistance—appears to be essential for the development of Alzheimer's disease.

Every cell in your body depends on glucose to supply its energy needs. Your brain cells are no different. Your brain cells are continually active, even while you are sleeping, so they have constant need for glucose. In Alzheimer's disease, the brain has lost its ability to properly absorb and utilize glucose for energy. As a consequence, brain cells gradually degenerate and die, leading to memory and cognitive loss. In essence, the brain has become insulin resistant. For this reason, Alzheimer's is considered a form of diabetes—brain diabetes—and is referred to as type 3 diabetes.[5]

Alzheimer's disease isn't the only neurodegenerative condition associated with insulin resistance. Studies of Parkinson's disease patients have also provided evidence for altered glucose metabolism and insulin resistance.[6] Since the 1950s, insulin resistance has been reported in a significant percentage of patients with amyotrophic lateral sclerosis (ALS), a fatal brain wasting disease that causes the death of neurons controlling voluntary muscles.[7-8]

Insulin Resistance and Obesity

Insulin resistance is a primary cause of obesity and overweight. Virtually everyone who is overweight is insulin resistant to some extent. Insulin resistance is present in anyone whose fasting blood sugar is 91 mg/dl (3.6 mmol/l) or more. Not only does insulin shuttle glucose into our cells, but it triggers the conversion of glucose into fat and shuttles fat into fat cells. Insulin is a fat storage hormone.

Whenever you eat carbohydrate, it is converted into glucose and released into the bloodstream. This triggers the release of insulin. If your pancreas is working properly, every time you eat carbohydrate, your blood glucose levels rise, followed by a rise in insulin levels. Elevated insulin shifts the body into a state of fat production and storage. This is what leads to weight gain. The more carbohydrate you eat, the more you are likely to store fat and gain weight.

Eating fat and protein does not significantly raise blood glucose levels; therefore, there is no corresponding rise in insulin and the body does not store fat. You don't gain weight eating fat and protein, unless you eat them with a source of carbohydrate. It is the carbohydrate that triggers the rise of glucose and insulin. The more carbohydrate calories you eat, the higher your insulin levels will rise and the greater the fat storage effect. You won't gain weight eating fat and protein with a modest amount of carbohydrate, especially if the source of carbohydrate is composed mostly of water, fiber, and nutrients like

34

zucchini, broccoli, asparagus, and other low-carb vegetables. Eating breads, cereals, potatoes, crackers, desserts, and sweets, which are high in sugar and starch, have the greatest effect on rising insulin levels and promoting weight gain.

Insulin resistance compounds the problem. If you are insulin resistant, your blood sugar and insulin levels are elevated 24 hours a day. Therefore, your body is in a metabolic state in which it is continually trying to store fat, even when you are not eating and even when you are sleeping. Since the body is trying to convert glucose into fat and store it away, it is very difficult to lose fat, even on an extremely low-calorie diet.

One of the reasons why the ketogenic diet is so effective as a means for weight loss is that it has little effect on blood glucose or insulin levels. Even though the majority of calories comes from fat, eating fat does not make you fat—carbohydrate does. Without carbohydrate in the diet, as in fasting or eating a ketogenic diet, the body pulls fat out of storage to supply much of its energy needs. Therefore, you lose weight.

THE MCT KETOGENIC DIET

The original or classic ketogenic diet was not without its drawbacks. The diet required a trained dietitian to teach parents how to properly prepare every meal and snack to the 4:1 or 3:1 ratio. As you might imagine, meals consisting of 90 percent fat were of limited appeal and quickly became tiresome. Many parents and patients found the diet too difficult to prepare and too unappetizing. Consequently, many could not keep with it long enough to achieve satisfactory results. As many as 20 percent could not tolerate the diet and failed to follow through with it. In 1938 a new anticonvulsant drug, phenytoin (Dilantin), was developed. Taking a pill was much easier than worrying about preparing and eating a specific diet. The focus of research quickly turned to discovering new drugs. The ketogenic diet was mostly ignored by researchers and was used primarily as a last resort to treat very serious cases that did not respond to drug therapy.

In the 1960s it was discovered that a certain group of fats known as medium chain triglycerides (MCTs) can be readily converted into ketones by the liver regardless of blood glucose levels or what other foods were consumed in the diet. Blood levels of ketones could be raised significantly simply by consuming a source of MCTs, without fasting or being on a ketogenic diet.

MCTs are found in only a few foods. By far the most abundant natural source of MCTs comes from coconut. Coconut oil is composed predominantly of MCTs. Simply consuming coconut oil raises blood ketone levels, even if the diet also contains carbohydrate. Combining coconut oil with a ketogenic diet raises blood ketones even higher and enhances the therapeutic effects of the diet.

Coconut oil consists of 63 percent MCTs. Researchers reasoned that if they could produce an oil with a higher MCT content, it would make the ketogenic diet even better. Through the process of distillation, the individual fatty acids in coconut oil can be separated and then recombined to produce an oil that is 100 percent MCTs. The resulting product is called *MCT oil*, also referred as *fractionated coconut oil*.

In 1971, Peter Huttenlocher developed a ketogenic diet in which about 60 percent of the calories came from MCT oil. This allowed more protein and three to four times as much carbohydrate as the classic ketogenic diet. Total fat consumption could be reduced from 90 percent of calories to about 70 percent (60 percent MCT, 10 percent other fats), with about 20 percent protein and 10 percent carbohydrate to round out the diet.

While some of the MCT oil was incorporated into the food, it was often consumed by mixing it with at least twice its volume of skimmed milk, chilled, and sipped during meals. Huttenlocher tested it on 12 children and adolescents with severe epilepsy with difficult-to-treat seizures. Most of the children improved in both seizure control and alertness, producing results that were similar to those of the classic ketogenic diet. The MCT ketogenic diet is considered more nutritious than the classic diet and allows patients the option to eat more protein and carbohydrate, providing a greater variety of foods and ways to prepare meals, making the diet much more palatable.

Despite all the positives with the MCT ketogenic diet, there were some drawbacks. Consuming too much MCT oil can cause nausea, vomiting, and diarrhea. Many patients have had to abandon the MCT ketogenic diet because they could not tolerate these side effects. A modified MCT ketogenic diet, which uses a combination of the MCTs and other fats, was found to be more tolerable and is currently being used in many hospitals.

Too much pure MCT oil is not tolerated well by many people, so other fats (known as *long chain triglycerides*, or LCTs) were added to ease the symptoms. Interestingly, unaltered coconut oil naturally contains 37 percent LCTs, thus accomplishing the same thing as combining MCTs with a source of LCTs. Coconut oil is much better tolerated than MCT oil and is much more versatile and useful in food preparation. A coconut oil-based ketogenic diet is just as effective as the modified MCT ketogenic diet.

THE MODIFIED ATKINS DIET

In the 1990s Dr. Robert Atkins published his bestselling book *Dr. Atkins' New Diet Revolution,* promoting a low-carb diet for weight loss and better health. He outlined four phases to his diet: the first and most restrictive phase limited total carbohydrate consumption to 20 grams a day (in comparison, the classic ketogenic diet restricts daily carbohydrate to 10 to 15 grams). This was an induction phase that was only meant to last a couple of weeks before moving on to phase two, where more carbohydrate could be consumed. There was no limit on the amount of fat or protein that could be eaten. In the initial phase of the diet, most people would get into a state of *ketosis*—a metabolic state in which the body burns more fat and ketones than glucose. When ketosis is induced by dietary means it is often referred to as nutritional ketosis. Ketones can be remarkably therapeutic and produce much of the beneficial effects of fasting. Most people can get into a mild state of nutritional ketosis by limiting total carbohydrate intake to 40 or 50 grams a day. Atkins encouraged those on the diet to get into ketosis. He taught that in the induction phase of his diet,entering ketosis is an indication that body fat is being dissolved and utilized to meet the body's daily energy needs. As body fat is burned for energy, weight is reduced. In this case, nutritional ketosis is a sign the body is losing its excess fat and weight.

Even though the induction phase of the Atkins diet does not produce as high a level of nutritional ketosis as the classic ketogenic diet, people reported that it controlled their seizures. In response to these accounts, researchers at Johns Hopkins Hospital put volunteers on the induction phase of the Atkins diet for extended periods of time, referring to it as a modified Atkins diet. The modified Atkins diet places no limit on calories or protein, and the lower overall ketogenic ratio (approximately 1:1) does not need to be consistently maintained in each meal of the day. Carbohydrates were initially limited to 10 grams per day in children, 15 grams per day in adults, and increased to 20-30 grams per day after a month or so, depending on the effect on seizure control. The researchers reported that the modified Atkins diet reduced seizure frequency by more than 50 percent in 43 percent of patients and by more than 90 percent in 27 percent of the patients.[9] This and other studies have shown that seizure control with the modified Atkins diet compares favorably with the classic ketogenic diet. Although a higher level of ketosis may provide slightly better protection against seizures, the lower level is still highly effective.

The ketogenic diet that is promoted today for weight loss and for overall improvement in health is a version of the modified Atkins ketogenic diet. Total carbohydrate intake is generally limited to no more than 30 grams per day, although some people consume a little more or less.

THE COCONUT KETOGENIC DIET

The classic and MCT ketogenic diets are difficult to follow because every gram of carbohydrate, protein, and fat must be calculated and served at each meal. The modified Atkins diet, which focuses primarily on carbohydrate intake, is much easier and allows greater flexibility and variety in foods. Atkins never mentioned the use of coconut oil, letting each individual choose the types of fat he or she preferred. Some people used predominately polyunsaturated fats, and others avoided adding much additional fat of any kind. However, eating too much polyunsaturated vegetable oils can become detrimental. The addition of coconut oil can significantly enhance the ketone production and the positive effects of the Atkins diet. Using coconut oil as the primary source of fat in a modified Atkins diet is sometimes referred to as the Coconut Ketogenic Diet.

Most people can show measurable ketones in their urine by restricting carbohydrate intake to 40 to 50 grams. This produces a mild ketogenic effect. However, limiting total carbohydrate to about 30 grams per day produces better results, yet still allows for plenty of dietary choices and options. In the beginning, you need to calculate every gram of carbohydrate you eat. This is very important. You do not want to estimate or guess, as this will decrease the effectiveness of the diet. As you gain experience, you will be able to prepare meals without actually calculating each gram of carbohydrate; a diet diary will be helpful in keeping track of carbohydrates in frequently eaten foods. For the first month or so you need to pay particular attention to stay strictly within your carbohydrate limit. After some experience, you will learn how to prepare and eat meals with about the right amount of carbohydrate to remain in ketosis.

Many ketogenic recipes in books and on the internet list the number of grams of carbohydrate, protein, and fat as well as calories per serving. Packaged foods list the amount of carbohydrate in the nutrition facts label on the container. This label lists both total carbohydrate and fiber content. Do not use total carbohydrate. You are interested in finding the amount of net carbohydrate (net carbs). This term refers to carbohydrate that is digestible, provides calories, and raises blood sugar. Dietary fiber is also a carbohydrate, but it does not raise blood sugar or supply calories, so it is not included. Most plant foods will contain both digestible carbohydrate and fiber. To calculate the net carbohydrate content, subtract the grams of fiber from the grams of total carbohydrate listed on the food label.

If you make your own meals from fresh ingredients, you can use a table of nutrient values to calculate the net carbs and other nutrients. An easy-to-use, open-access nutrient chart listing fresh produce, grains, meats, and dairy can be accessed at www.coconutresearchcenter.org (look under the heading "Ketogenic Diet"). A good nutrient calculator with data on both fresh and processed foods can be accessed for free at www.calorieking.com. An excellent calculator available for a reasonable fee is www.carbmanager.com.

In order to stay under your carbohydrate limit for the day, you will want to eliminate or dramatically reduce all high-carb foods in your diet. For instance, a slice of white bread contains 12 grams of carbohydrate. Just two slices will bring you close to your 30 gram limit. Since all vegetables and fruits contain carbohydrate, you would be restricted to eating only meat and fat for the rest of the day in order to stay under your limit, which is not a good idea. A single medium-size baked potato contains 32 grams of carbohydrate—more than a day's allotment. An apple has 18 grams, an orange 12 grams, and a medium-size banana 25 grams. Breads and grains contain the highest amount of carbohydrate. A single 4-inch (10 cm) pancake without any syrup or sweeteners has 13 grams, a 10-inch (27 cm) tortilla has 34 grams, and a plain bagel has 57 grams. Candy and desserts are just as high in carbohydrate and provide almost no nutritional value, so they should be completely eliminated from the diet. All breads and most fruits are very limited if not totally eliminated.

Vegetables, however, are much lower in carbohydrate. One cup of asparagus has 2 grams, a cup of raw cabbage 2 grams, and a cup of cauliflower 2.5 grams. All types of lettuce are very low in carbohydrate: a cup of shredded lettuce has only about 0.5 gram.

You can easily fill up on green salad and other low-carb vegetables without worrying too much about going over your carbohydrate limit.

Although fruit normally is fairly high in carbohydrate, a limited amount can be consumed. Fruits with the lowest carbohydrate content are berries such as blackberries (½ cup contains 3.5 grams of carbohydrate), boysenberries (½ cup contains 4.5 grams), raspberries (½ cup contains 3 grams), and strawberries (½ cup, sliced, contains 4.5 grams). Any fruit, vegetable, or even grain product can be eaten, as long as the portion size is not so big that it puts you over your carbohydrate limit. Since most fruits, starchy vegetables, and grains are high in carbohydrate, it is best to simply avoid them altogether.

High protein foods need to be limited because the body can convert about half of the protein you eat into glucose, with all the adverse effects associated with it. As a rule of thumb, protein intake should be limited to about 1.2 grams for every 1 kg (2.2 lb) of normal or desirable body weight. This amounts to limiting your protein intake to about 60 to 90 grams per day, depending on your size and level of physical activity. The smaller and less active you are, the less you need. Athletes can eat a little more. A 3 ounce (85 g) steak, which is about the size of a deck of playing cards, contains 21 grams of protein. A 3 ounce chicken breast contains 26 grams of protein. The chicken supplies more protein because beef contains more fat and less protein. Fatty fish, such as cod, contains 19 grams of protein per 3 ounce serving.

Most fresh meats, fish, and fowl are essentially carbohydrate-free. Eggs and cheese contain very small amounts. Processed meats, however, often contain sugar or other fillers as well as preservatives and other food additives. Processed meats include lunch meats, bacon, ham, sausage, and such. They often contain sugar, preservatives, flavor enhancers and other additives, so you must read the ingredient and nutrition facts labels carefully.

There is no limitation on fat intake, particularly saturated and monounsaturated fats, and they should used freely as they are providing most of your energy in the absence of carbohydrate. You are encouraged to use as much fat as possible in meal preparation. Forget the lean cuts of meat! Eat fatty meats and eat all the fat, including the skin on chicken and other fowl. Eat all the meat drippings after cooking. Add more fat when possible. The added fat makes foods taste better. You will be surprised how good vegetables taste when they are smothered in meat drippings, butter, or coconut oil. If you weren't a fan of vegetables before, you will become a veggie-lover now that you can spruce them up with fat.

A person can live on this diet indefinitely. It provides all the nutrients needed for good health. However, when in ketosis the body seems to use up electrolytes at a faster pace. A sign of low electrolyte levels is muscle cramps, especially leg cramps during the night—a fairly common occurrence for those following a ketogenic diet. For this reason, it is beneficial to include an additional source of magnesium, potassium, and sodium in the diet. Magnesium and potassium can be added with a daily mineral supplement: 250 to 300 mg of magnesium and 99 mg of potassium daily is generally adequate. Sodium is best taken by using a liberal amount of sea salt in food preparation. Don't be afraid of using salt. While you are in ketosis, salt in food will not adversely affect blood pressure. In fact, if you are following the diet correctly, your blood pressure will actually improve.

KETOSIS MONITORING

Many people make the mistake of thinking that if they eat a lot of protein and fat and few vegetables, they are eating keto. Big mistake! After eating this way for awhile they may wonder why they are not experiencing all the benefits others have when they have gone keto. They may even give up and claim the ketogenic diet didn't work for them. The problem was not the ketogenic diet, but rather a failure to follow the diet properly. If the diet does not get you into ketosis, then it is not a ketogenic diet. It may be a high-protein diet, or a low-carb diet, or something else, but it is not a ketogenic diet.

Often people read an article or two on the ketogenic diet and want to try it, but instead of taking the time and effort to actually count the number of carbs they eat, they just make an estimate and hope they are close. Estimates are usually way off. We tend to underestimate the amount of carbs and protein in our foods and overestimate the amount of fat. One of the problems is that fat supplies twice as many calories as either protein or carbohydrate. You cannot eyeball it, judging by size or volume alone. When you first start going keto you must calculate the number of grams of carbs, protein, and fat you eat at each meal. This is important so that you can get an accurate idea of the volume of food you can eat. After a few weeks of doing this, you will gain a sense of how much you can eat and more accurately estimate meal portions. Without this experience, accurate estimation is virtually impossible. Also, over time people commonly tend to drift by increasing protein and carb intake and reducing fat intake until they are no longer eating keto.

Once a ketogenic diet is started, it takes a few days for blood levels of ketones to build up. As the liver's store of glucose (glycogen) is depleted, ketone production shifts into high gear. After three or four days, you will be able to measure the relative amount of ketones in the blood using a urine ketosis test strip, also known as a lipolysis test strip.

One end of the test strip is dipped into a fresh specimen of urine. The strip changes color depending on the ketone concentration in the urine. The urine test measures the amount of acetoacetate present. With the test strip a person can tell if his or her blood ketone level is "none," "trace," "small," "moderate," or "large." The test is helpful in that it indicates if the dietary changes are producing ketones and to what degree. As you add more carbohydrate into the diet, ketone levels drop. To increase ketosis you can reduce carbohydrate consumption.

The urine test strips are the cheapest and easiest method for testing ketone levels. Ketosis test strips are sold in most pharmacies. Two other methods of testing ketone levels include a blood monitor and a breath analyzer. Both provide more precise measurements, but are much more expensive. You really don't need these types of monitoring devices, the urine strips provide all the information you need to tell if and when you are in ketosis and to what degree.

4

Traditional Diets

NUTRITION AND PHYSICAL DEGENERATION

In ages past, infections, starvation, and trauma were the major causes of ill health and death. Today it is chronic, degenerative diseases, many of which were rare or unheard of among our ancestors. The very first recorded heart attack death was reported in the 1876. It was such a rare occurrence at the time that it was described in a medical journal. Coronary heart disease remained a very rare occurrence until the 1920s, when heart attack deaths began to skyrocket. By 1950, coronary heart disease had become the number one cause of death in America. Obesity in the US has tripled over the past 40 years and diabetes has increased by 700 percent. Alzheimer's disease wasn't even recognized until 1906. The incidence of cancer, arthritis, glaucoma, asthma, and other chronic diseases have likewise skyrocketed over the past 100 years. These diseases were rare among our ancestors and are still generally unseen among many indigenous societies still following their traditional diets and ways of life.. These once uncommon chronic diseases are often referred to as diseases of modern civilization.

Doctors often blame our increased lifespan for these diseases, saying modern medicine and improved nutrition has allowed people to live longer, so now we are developing degenerative diseases more frequently than was seen in the past. However, chronic disease doesn't just affect the elderly, in fact, chronic disease is occurring at younger and younger ages. It is not unusual for cancer, arthritis, and other degenerative diseases to strike people in their 30s or even younger. Also, even a century or two ago many people lived into their 90s. Most of these people continued to work in the fields and remained physically active and relatively healthy until they died—a far cry from today when people are confined to rest homes and care facilities, where they often require constant medical care and supervision for the last several years of their lives.

Modern food processing started around the beginning of the 20th century. Before that time, most of our food came from local farms. The rise in chronic disease over the past century corresponds exactly with this dramatic change in diet and lifestyle. Instead of eating mostly whole freshly grown or fermented foods, we began eating highly processed, refined, packaged foods. White refined flour and polished rice replaced whole wheat and brown rice. Sugar consumption in the US increased from about 15 pounds per person per year in 1800 to 152 pounds by 1999. Traditional fats like lard, butter, and coconut oil were replaced by more modern and highly processed vegetable oils (corn, soybean, canola, safflower, etc.). The process of hydrogenating vegetable oils for the manufacture of shortening and margarine first appeared in 1911. Fresh meat and produce was replaced by prepared meals loaded with preservatives, dyes, flavor enhancers and other chemicals, then packaged in cans, bottles, boxes, and freezer bags. In just a few decades our entire way of eating changed.

Despite a slurry of wonder drugs and the miracle of modern medicine, we may live a little longer on average than our ancestors, but these extra years are not healthy, happy, disease-free years, but years of degeneration, incapacitation, and constant medical care that just manages to keep us breathing, but not much else.

This pattern has been documented throughout the world. Many accounts from scientists, explorers, and missionaries traveling to the far reaches of the globe describe indigenous people who were generally robust and healthy, with excellent physical development and free of deformity. However, as modern processed foods were introduced, their health and appearance began to decline.

The link between the rise of degenerative disease and diet was aptly demonstrated back in the 1930s by Weston A. Price, DDS (1870-1948). Dr. Price served as the Chairman of the Research Section of the American Dental Association from 1914-1923 and is noted for his extensive research on nutrition and dental health.

During his long career as a practicing dentist, he observed an increasing incidence of tooth decay, gum disease, dental deformities, and other health problems late in his career that were rare in his earlier years. He was seeing more and more children with narrow dental arches and crowded teeth. When the wisdom teeth erupted, there often wasn't room for them, which required that they be extracted. This was a curious phenomenon because early in his career patients rarely had to have wisdom teeth removed. Remains of ancient humans show broad dental arches and healthy wisdom teeth. It didn't make sense that the human body, as perfectly designed as it was, would suddenly grow teeth that didn't work and required surgical removal. At no time in human history had there been a need to remove wisdom teeth from so many people. It wasn't just the teeth, he noticed that the general health of his patients were declining; they were developing degenerative diseases at an increasing rate. He was seeing the so-called diseases of "old age" in younger and younger patients.

Price was a firsthand witness to the transformation and revolution of modern food processing. He wondered if the changes in the diet were related to the decline in health he was witnessing. He set out to find the answer. The way he planned to do this was to compare healthy populations who subsisted on traditional diets with those who had incorporated modern processed foods into their diets. To avoid other influences that may affect health, the people studied would be of the same genetic background and live in the same geographic area. The only difference would be the diet.

Today it is nearly impossible to find a population that relies solely on traditional foods. Modern foods are found virtually everywhere throughout the world. But in the 1930s there were still many populations that subsisted primarily on their ancestral foods without modern influences.

Dr. Price spent nearly a decade traveling around the world locating and studying these populations. He traveled to isolated valleys in the Swiss Alps, the Outer and Inner Hebrides off the coast of Scotland, and Inuit villages in Alaska, and visited American Indians in central and northern Canada, the Melanesians and Polynesians on numerous islands throughout the South Pacific, tribes in eastern and central Africa, the Aborigines of Australia, Malay tribes on islands north of Australia, the Maori of New Zealand, and South American Indians in Peru and the Amazon Basin.

When Dr. Price visited an area, he would examine the people's health, particularly their teeth, and made careful note of the foods they ate and meticulously analyzed the nutritional content of the diet. Samples of the food were sent to his laboratory, where detailed analyses were made. It didn't take long for him to notice the contrast in health between those who lived entirely on indigenous foods and those who had incorporated modern foods into their diets.

Wherever he found people living on traditional foods, he noted that both their dental and physical health were in excellent condition, but when the people began eating modern processed foods, their health quickly declined. In the absence of modern medical care, physical degeneration was pronounced. Dental diseases, as well as infectious and degenerative diseases such as arthritis and tuberculosis, were common among those eating Western foods.

He also found that it didn't take a dramatic change in the diet for degenerative disease to begin to creep in. Simply adding a few commercial products, which displaced more nutritious foods, was all that was needed. The most common imported foods were white flour, sugar, vegetable oils, and canned goods.

One of the things he noted was that parents who began adding modern foods into their diet gave birth to children whose teeth and bone structure were slightly malformed. The dental arch became narrowed, teeth became crowded, and wisdom teeth became impacted. In contrast, those people whose parents ate traditional foods had excellent dental health and development. They possessed wide dental arches with straight, healthy teeth and their wisdom teeth came in without problems.

The same degeneration in health that was occurring in these isolated societies when they adopted modern foods was the same that he had been seeing in his dental practice. The connection was obvious. Modern processed foods were nutritionally deficient, and as a consequence, people were developing a greater number of degenerative conditions and children were being born with developmental deficiencies. Dr. Price's findings were published in

1939 in a book titled *Nutrition and Physical Degeneration*. This book, which is still in print and currently in its eighth edition, is considered a classic in nutritional science.

Chronic degenerative diseases are rare among societies that live on traditional diets consisting of whole, natural foods. When populations are introduced to modern civilization and adopt Western foods, diseases of modern civilization begin to develop. Dr. Price found that within just a single generation, these cultures began to experience degenerative diseases, clearly indicating that they are not caused by genetics.

Price also observed that the types of foods eaten varied greatly from one population to the next. Inuit and Canadian Indians ate a diet that consisted almost entirely of meat and fat. The Pacific Islanders consumed large quantities of fruit, root vegetables, and fat (primarily from coconuts). The inhabitants of the islands off the coast of Scotland subsisted largely on oats and seafood. Those in the Swiss Alps relied primarily on dairy and never ate fish. Despite the wide variety in their diets, the one thing they did have in common was that the foods were fresh or fermented, relatively whole, and minimally processed. There was no highly processed sugar or refined white flour. All fats were natural, consisting predominantly of saturated fats derived from meat, dairy, or coconut. They used no polyunsaturated vegetable oils. The small quantity of honey or sugarcane some populations may have eaten was seasonal and constituted only a tiny part of their overall diet.

ANCESTRAL DIETS

Recognizing diet as a primary cause of chronic disease, many people have adopted a more natural diet. Some people have returned to eating the way people did in the past, consuming only foods that were eaten by our ancestors. Such diets are referred to as ancestral diets.

The most popular ancestral diet right now is the Paleo diet. Those following this diet try to eat only foods that were available to our Paleolithic ancestors that lived some 10,000 to 20,000 years ago. The Weston A. Price Foundation, an organization based on the discoveries of Dr. Price, promotes an ancestral diet, but does not go so far back in history. This diet encourages the consumption of organically produced whole, natural foods, much like the foods our great-grandmother would have eaten. A similar diet is the ethnic ancestral diet in which people eat the types of foods their own direct ancestors ate. For example, there are native Hawaiians that eat only traditional Hawaiian foods such as poi, taro root, plantains, coconut, breadfruit, fish, and so forth.

While there are slight differences in the types of foods eaten between these ancestral diets, the one thing they all have in common is the avoidance of modern processed foods. Ancestral diets tend to avoid foods or food ingredients that would have been unrecognizable to our ancestors such as soda, candy, chips, processed lunch meats, and foods that contain artificial or chemical ingredients like MSG or aspartame. Foods are organically grown and definitely do not contain any genetically modified ingredients. Processed sugars of all types are also avoided. In essence, the foods eaten are those that would be recognized by our ancestors or that would be available to them in their day.

We have become fat and sick from our modern foods. If we want to regain our health we need to eat like our ancestors did by consuming fresh, natural foods. If you start fasting or go on a ketogenic diet to overcome some health problem, yet continue to eat highly processed foods, refined grains, and sugar, you will not be successful. The keto diet and fasting may give you some relief, but as soon as you start eating poorly again, your health problems will return. You cannot expect to be free from chronic poor health as long as you continue to eat the same types of foods that caused the problems in the first place.

ULTRA-PROCESSED FOODS SHORTEN YOUR LIFE

When you go to the grocery store, you normally find a relatively small section where they sell fresh produce and another selling fresh meats, while the vast majority of the space in the store is dedicated to selling packaged, boxed, canned, and frozen foods. Most of these are in the form of snacks, desserts, and ready-to-eat meals or heat-and-serve meals. Almost all of these products have undergone extensive processing and are designed to have a long shelf life. According to the NOVA food classification system used in research, these are called ultra-processed foods. They are defined as those manufactured industrially from multiple ingredients that usually include additives used for technological and/or cosmetic purposes. Such foods are high in additives, unhealthy fats, and refined starches and sugars, and are poor sources of protein, dietary fiber, and micronutrients. Generally, any processed, packaged food that contains more than three or four ingredients would be considered ultra-processed.

One of the characteristics of ultra-processing is the addition of food additives. These ingredients are used to enhance the flavor, texture, and appearance of the food, and extend shelf life. While some additives are derived from herbs and other natural sources, most are industrially produced chemical products such as monosodium glutamate (MSG), aspartame, hydrogenated vegetable oils, sodium nitrate, butylated hydroxytoluene (BHT), butylhydroxyanisol (BHA), and tert-butylhydroquinone (TBHQ), to name a few. In addition to ingredients that are purposely added, there are those that find their way into foods by accident or as a consequence of processing and are not listed in the ingredient label. These include pesticides, antibiotics, growth hormones, fecal material, bacteria and mold, plastic, dirt and grease, and detergent and disinfectant residue from processing equipment. More and more genetically modified corn, soy, canola, and other GMOs are also finding their way into our foods.

Few, if any, of these additives could be considered healthy or even benign, most are toxic. Although recognized as potentially harmful, they are not considered a health hazard because the amount of each one in any given product is so small, it is believed to pose little danger. That might be true if only one chemical was added and if you didn't eat any other foods with chemical additives, but most processed products have multiple questionable additives and such foods are eaten at nearly every meal. This greatly increases the amount of the toxins ingested. Also, the toxicity of these chemicals can be greatly increased when consumed in combination so that the toxic effects work synergistically, making the combination more toxic then when they are consumed individually. When consumed every day, day in and day out, the toxic effects can be accumulative and manifest themselves as chronic health problems.

In addition to toxic food additives, most of the foods in our diet are nutrient deficient. Few people nowadays make their meals from basic ingredients—meat, eggs, dairy, fruit, vegetables, whole grains/flour, herbs, and spices. It is far easier and quicker to buy something that requires little or no preparation before eating. In his research, Weston A. Price found that the first and most common products introduced into underdeveloped societies were sugar and refined white flour. He noted that it didn't take much of these to have a significant impact on the health of the population. The people may have maintained their normal native diets for the most part, but with just the addition of a little sugar and white flour, their health declined rapidly. The displacement of their normal nourishing foods with nutrient deficient, highly processed carbohydrates led to nutrient deficiencies and physical degeneration.

Food processing and refining removes and destroys many nutrients. Sugar, for example, has a total of zero vitamins and minerals. But it does contain fattening calories. White flour, likewise, has been stripped of its vitamin and mineral rich bran and germ, leaving almost pure starch. Starch is nothing more than sugar (glucose). White rice is the same: during processing, the vitamin-rich bran is removed, leaving the white starchy portion behind. Excessive consumption of sugar and refined starch is a primary cause of insulin resistance and diabetes.

For the most part, our typical diet consists of foods which are mostly empty calories. Few of us eat enough fruits and vegetables. When we do consume them, it's generally as condiments—pickles and lettuce on a sandwich, tomato sauce and onions on a pizza. Our food is loaded with calories, but nutritionally deficient. The consequence is that you can eat and eat and eat until you are overweight, yet still be malnourished.

According to the World Health Organization, 70 to 80 percent of people in developed nations die from lifestyle- or diet-caused diseases. The majority of cancers are caused by what we put into our bodies. Heart disease, stroke, and atherosclerosis, the biggest killers in affluent nations, are dietary diseases. Diabetes is a diet-related disease. Numerous studies have shown that vitamins, minerals, and other nutrients in foods protect us from these degenerative diseases.

When we think of malnutrition, we usually think of emaciated drought victims in Africa or starving people in Asia. In more affluent countries, the problem is more subtle. Symptoms of malnutrition are not as evident. Overweight people don't look malnourished, and methods of diagnosing deficiency diseases require malnutrition to be in an advanced stage before they can be detected.

When a variety of foods are available, few people develop obvious symptoms of malnutrition like scurvy or beriberi, even when their diets are nutritionally poor. Instead, they suffer from *subclinical malnutrition*. Subclinical malnutrition is a condition in which a person consumes just enough essential nutrients to prevent full-blown symptoms of severe malnutrition, but the body is still nutrient deficient and prone to slow, premature degeneration. This condition can go on unnoticed indefinitely. In Western countries the problem of subclinical malnutrition is epidemic. Our foods are sadly depleted of nutrients. We eat, and even overeat, but may still be malnourished because our foods do not contain all the essential nutrients our bodies need to function optimally. As a result, the immune system is chronically depressed, the body cannot fight off infections well, and tissues and cells starving for nutrients slowly degenerate.

Growing evidence indicates that higher intake of ultra-processed foods is associated with a higher incidence of chronic and degenerative disease and early death. Studies have found that the consumption of ultra-processed foods is associated with higher rates of obesity, insulin resistance, metabolic syndrome, high blood pressure and elevated LDL cholesterol levels, all of which can increase the risk of early death.[1-2]

A recent study published in *JAMA International Medicine* evaluated the relationship between overall mortality risk and the consumption of ultra-processed foods. The study conducted by researchers from health institutions in France examined nearly 45,000 adults age 45 and older for two years. The study analyzed the subjects' diet and health status. They found that ultra-processed foods comprised a mean of over 29 percent of the calories in the participants' diet. Not surprisingly, the more ultra-processed foods consumed, the greater their body mass index. They also evaluated deaths and calculated a 14 percent higher risk of early death for each 10 percent increase in ultra-processed foods consumed.[3]

Ultra-processed foods account for 36 percent of the total calories consumed by children and adults in France, 48 percent in Canada, and 58 percent in the US. The *JAMA* study on French adults over the age of 45 showed a lower consumption rate for older adults than for the general French population. A number of studies have shown that younger people are more likely to consume ultra-processed foods, making them more susceptible to degenerative disease in the future. This may be one of the reasons why chronic diseases that were once considered a consequence of aging are occurring at increasingly younger ages.

Consuming organic foods is a preferable option as it eliminates many questionable additives, GMOs, and chemicals used in agriculture. However, there are many packaged, prepared organic "health foods" that would still be classified as ultra-processed. The best choice is unprocessed or minimally processed food, which is organically grown, just like the foods our ancestors ate.

DIETARY FATS
Traditional Fats

One of the most important foods in your diet is fat. Fat is an essential nutrient. Our ancestors highly prized fat and recognized its importance in achieving good health. They wasted none of the fat in the game they caught, collecting every morsel of fat from behind the eyeballs and around the kidneys and other organs, even taking the time and effort to crack open the bones to harvest the fatty bone morrow. Pregnant and nursing women were given extra portions of fat to ensure the health of both the mother and child. Fat contributed between 50 to 90 percent of the calories in the diet of our hunter-gatherer ancestors. Fat has been a part of the human diet for many thousands of years. As a result, our bodies are well adapted to metabolizing fat—particularly saturated fat.

Prior to the 20th century the fats and oils most commonly used throughout the world were animal fats and fruit oils (palm, coconut, and olive oils). Lard was the most commonly used fat in most countries. These oils were used because they are relatively easy to produce. Lard and beef tallow could be separated simply by heating. Animal fats and fruit oils are rich sources of saturated and monounsaturated fats. In 1909, 82 percent of the fat in our diet was of animal origin. Most of the remainder was from fruit oils.

Polyunsaturated vegetable oils or seed oils derived from seeds or grains were less frequently used at this time because most of them required greater effort to extract and process. Another problem is that they are more unstable than the saturated and monounsaturated fats and go rancid quickly when exposed to heat, light, and oxygen. For this reason, they were not generally used for food until after the invention of the hydraulic oil press in the latter part of the 19th century, as they could then be produced quickly and cheaply.

Types of Fats

Fat is one of the three energy-producing macronutrients in our diet, along with protein and carbohydrate. Fats are composed of fat molecules known as fatty acids. There are many different types of fatty acids. All of them are composed of a chain of carbon atoms, each attached to two hydrogen atoms. You can classify the fatty acids into three separate categories depending on the degree of saturation: saturated, monounsaturated, and polyunsaturated. Saturation refers to how many pairs of hydrogen atoms each fatty acid contains. A fatty acid that contains the maximum number of hydrogen atoms it can possible hold is said to be saturated with hydrogen. A monounsaturated fatty acid has room for one pair of hydrogen atoms and a polyunsaturated fatty acid has room for two or more pairs of hydrogen atoms.

Fatty acids come in different sizes. The exact number of hydrogen atoms is determined by the size of the fatty acid or the length of its carbon chain. The vast majority of the fatty acids in our diet have a chain length of 14 to 22 carbon atoms long. These are known as long chain fatty acids (LCFAs). Those with chain lengths of between 6 and 12 carbons are known as medium chain fatty acids (MCFAs), and those with less than 6 are referred to as short chain fatty acids (SCFAs). The degree of saturation and length of each fatty acid influences how it is metabolized and utilized by the body. Therefore, the physiological effects of one fatty acid may be distinctly different from another. All of them can and are used by cells as fuel to produce energy, but they have other purposes as well, both structural and physiological.

The degree of saturation profoundly affects the chemical stability of fatty acids. The more unsaturated the fatty acid, the more unstable it is and the more easily it can oxidize or degrade and become rancid. Rancidity causes the production of highly destructive peroxide free radicals that can be harmful to living tissue. Fats can become oxidized either before or after consumption. Saturated fatty acids are very resistant to oxidation and rancidity and make excellent cooking oils. Polyunsaturated fatty acids are highly vulnerable to oxidation. Monounsaturated fatty acids are in between.

When fats are exposed to heat, light, or oxygen, they begin to oxidize. Polyunsaturated fats oxidize easily. Consequently, they go rancid quickly after being extracted from their source (seeds and grains) and degrade rapidly when exposed to heat, especially the heat used in cooking, so they do not make suitable cooking oils. Vegetable oils that contain a high percentage of polyunsaturated fatty acids include soybean, corn, safflower, sunflower, sesame, peanut, and canola—some of the most common so-called cooking oils. Food manufacturers aware of the rancidity problem with polyunsaturated vegetable oils have traditionally used butter, lard, coconut oil, and other predominantly saturated fats in food preparation, as they allow the foods to remain fresh and preserve their taste and texture longer than other fats.

The process of hydrogenation was invented to transform liquid vegetable oils into hardened fats resembling animal fats. Hydrogenation bombards polyunsaturated fatty acids with hydrogen atoms, causing them to become more saturated. As a consequence, they become more chemically stable and resistant to oxidation and rancidity. For this reason, cheap hydrogenated vegetable oils often replaced more expensive saturated fats in food production. Unfortunately, unnatural trans fatty acids are formed during the hydrogenation process. Trans fatty acids are fats that have an unnatural chemical configuration that doesn't allow them to be used or function like normal fatty acids, thus promoting cellular dysfunction that can lead to numerous health problems, including heart disease.

Hydrogenated vegetable oils were introduced into the United States in 1911 in the form of shortening and later as margarine. They were eventually used by food manufacturers and restaurants in place of saturated fats because they were mistakenly believed to

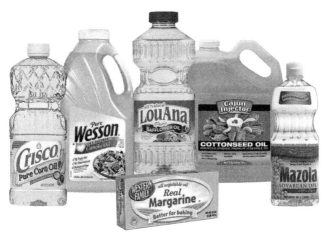

Ultra-processed vegetable oils rich in polyunsaturated fatty acids.

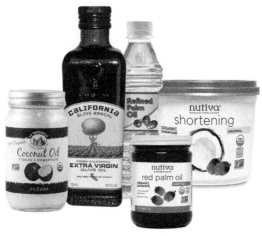

Traditional vegetable oils rich in monounsaturated and saturated fatty acids.

be a healthier option. Fortunately, the use of hydrogenated vegetable oils is on the decline as research has now clearly demonstrated their destructive nature.

When talking about fats you may hear the term *triglyceride*. The fatty acids in our foods are in the form of triglycerides, which are simply three fatty acids joined together by a glycerol molecule. The fat you see in meat and the oil you see in a bottle are in the form of triglycerides. When consumed, the triglycerides are broken down into individual fatty acids.

Fat Is a Vital Nutrient

Fat is the primary component of the ketogenic diet. It provides calories to replace calories from carbohydrate and protein, allowing you to have the energy to function normally and to even exercise or do physically demanding work. It supplies essential nutrients to keep you healthy and promote health and detoxification. Also, it provides bulk to satisfy hunger and ward off the food cravings that make dieting so arduous.

Dietary fat serves many important functions in the body. Some fats are so critical, such as linoleic and alpha-linolenic acids, that they are known as *essential fatty acids*—they cannot be made by the body so it is essential that they be included in the diet. An essential fatty acid deficiency can lead to many serious symptoms, including the following:

Dry and pale skin
Scaly dermatitis
Irregular or quilted appearance of the skin
Thick or cracked calluses
Weak or brittle fingernails
Dry or brittle hair
Hair loss
Dry eyes and mouth
Kidney dysfunction
High blood pressure
Numbness of the extremities
Joint swelling
Gastrointestinal distress
Immune dysfunction
Elevated LDL cholesterol
Atherosclerosis

Some fatty acids are considered conditionally essential, meaning they are critical during specific stages of life. For example, three medium chain fatty acids (caprylic, capric, and lauric acids) are essential during infancy. For this reason, they are found in human breast milk. In fact, they are found in the milk of all mammals for they are just as critical for these animals as they are for humans. All three of these are saturated fats. They are essential for infants because they serve the following roles:

• Protect against systemic infections

MCFAs possess potent antimicrobial properties that give them the power to kill disease-causing bacteria, viruses, and fungi. Infants are born with an underdeveloped immune system, which makes them highly vulnerable to systemic infection. The MCFAs in mother's milk provide a degree of protection against infectious illnesses.

• Establish a healthy gut microbiome

Many of the microorganisms that are vulnerable to the deadly effects of MCFAs are those that can inhabit the digestive tract and cause digestive disturbances, plaguing a person for life. Fortunately, MCFAs do not harm friendly gut bacteria that are essential for good digestive function and health. They kill the troublemakers but leave the good guys alone. Therefore, they are essential in establishing a healthy gut microbiome in the infant.

• Promote the proper development of the intestinal tract

MCFAs are absorbed into our cells very easily. They do not need the help of insulin or any special enzymes and therefore provide a quick and easy source of nutrition for the cells lining the intestinal tract. An infant's digestive tract is not completely developed when born. MCFAs provide the nutrition the cells need to quickly grow and mature properly so that the intestines function as they should.

• Train the immune system to mount a healthy defense against infections

MCFAs can train the infant's immune system to quickly recognize potential danger and mount an appropriate and effective defense. For example, *Staphylococcus aureus* is a bacterium that commonly inhabits the skin and sinuses. If it gets into the bloodstream, however, it can cause a serious infection. If the organism finds its way into the digestive tract, contact with a MCFA will kill it, causing the organism's outer membrane to break apart and fragment. A small fragment of this membrane can possibly be absorbed into the intestinal wall and find its way into the bloodstream. Here, the membrane fragment is identified as a foreign invader and a mild immune response in initiated that draws in white blood cells to destroy the fragment. Since the fragment is from a dead bacterium and is not a living organism, it poses no risk of infection and is quickly cleansed from the body. In this manner, the infant's body is trained to identify and quickly respond to potentially harmful organisms in the bloodstream.

• Provide a source of ketones, which are critical to normal brain development

After ingestion, many of the MCFAs are converted into ketones. Ketones are one of the two primary sources of energy used by the brain. When ketones enter the brain, they activate special proteins in the brain that regulate brain cell function, repair, and protection and stimulate brain cell synthesis. Ketones also provide the brain with the basic lipid building blocks necessary to make new brain cells. Infants' brains are rapidly growing for the first year or so after birth. They need ketones—the building blocks for brain cells—in order to grow and develop properly.

While these medium chain fatty acids are critical for infants, they are highly beneficial for adults as well. These fatty acids are found in only a small number of commonly eaten foods. By far the richest natural source of medium chain fatty acids is coconut oil. Coconut oil is composed of 63 percent medium chain fatty acids. The second most abundant source is palm kernel oil, containing 53 percent. The third richest source is dairy butter, consisting of 8 percent. Cream, milk, cheese, and other dairy products have smaller amounts. Although MCFAs are not "essential" for adults, they do provide substantial health benefits, including all of those listed above for infants. All medium chain fatty acids are saturated fats.

Fat serves many other important functions in the body. It supplies a vital source of energy for the body. It is necessary for proper growth, repair, and maintenance of body tissues. Every cell in your body is encased in a membrane that is composed of a double layer of fat molecules (phospholipids), most of which are made of saturated and monounsaturated fatty acids. The fat in our bodies consists of about 45 percent saturated, 50 percent monounsaturated, and only about 5 percent polyunsaturated fat. Consequently, the body's need for dietary saturated and monounsaturated fatty acids is much greater than for polyunsaturated fatty acids. Your body's need for saturated fat is nearly 10 times greater than its need for polyunsaturated fatty acids. While saturated and monounsaturated fatty acids can be synthesized in the body from other nutrients, we cannot make enough to satisfy our needs, so they must be included in our diet to achieve and maintain good health.[4-5]

Saturated fats are the preferred source of energy for the heart muscle and are essential for good lung function. They help protect the unsaturated fats in our bodies from the destructive action of free radicals, thus preventing much of the harm caused by lipid peroxidation, including the oxidation of cholesterol that has been linked to atherosclerosis and heart disease. They increase the production of HDL—the good cholesterol that protects against heart disease. They also increase the production of large buoyant LDL—another good cholesterol that is used to make hormones, including estrogen, progesterone, testosterone, and vitamin D, and is used as a structural component in cell membranes and as a covering on the axons of neurons to aid in cell-to-cell communication for proper brain and nerve function.

Fats are supernutrients. They are the source of many critically important fat soluble nutrients including vitamins A, D, E, and K, as well as beta-carotene, alpha-carotene, gamma-carotene, lycopene, lutein, and CoQ10. These nutrients are only found in the fatty portion of animal and vegetable foods.

Fats slow down the movement of food through the stomach and digestive system. This is important because it allows more time for foods to bathe in stomach acids and digestive enzymes. As a consequence, more nutrients are released from our foods and absorbed into the body, especially minerals which are normally tightly bound to other compounds. Fats improve the availability and absorption of almost all vitamins and minerals, including the water soluble vitamins and amino acids (protein).

Low-fat diets are actually detrimental because they prevent complete digestion of food and limit nutrient absorption, promoting mineral deficiencies. Calcium, for example, needs fat for proper absorption. For this reason, low-fat diets encourage osteoporosis. It is interesting that we often avoid fat as much as possible and eat low fat foods, including non-fat and low-fat milk, to get calcium—yet by eating reduced fat milks, the calcium is not effectively absorbed. This may be one of the reasons why people can drink loads of milk and take calcium supplements by the handful but still suffer from osteoporosis. Likewise, many vegetables are good sources of calcium. However, in order to take advantage of that calcium, you need to eat them with butter and cream or other foods that contain fat.

Many of the fat-soluble vitamins function as antioxidants that protect you from free-radical damage. By reducing the amount of fat in your diet, you limit the amount of protective antioxidant nutrients available to protect you from destructive free-radical reactions. Low-fat diets speed the process of degeneration and aging. This may be one of the reasons why those people who stay on very low-fat diets for any length of time often look pale and sickly.

Carotenoids are fat-soluble nutrients found in fruits and vegetables. The best known is beta-carotene. All of the carotenoids are known for their antioxidant capability. Many studies have shown them and other fat-soluble antioxidants to provide protection from degenerative disease and support immune system function.

Vegetables like broccoli and carrots have beta-carotene, but if you don't eat any oil with them you won't get the full benefit of the fat-soluble vitamins they contain. You can eat fruits and vegetables loaded with antioxidants and other nutrients, but if you don't include fat with them then you will only absorb a very small portion of these vital nutrients. Taking vitamin tablets won't help much because they too need fat to facilitate proper absorption. Eating a low-fat diet, therefore, can actually be detrimental.

So, if you want to get all the nutrients you can from the vegetables you eat, you need to add fat to them. Eating vegetables without added fat is in effect the same as eating a nutritionally poor meal. Adding a good source of fat in the diet is important in order to gain the most nutrition from your foods.

Saturated Fat Does Not Promote Heart Disease

Reducing dietary saturated fat has generally been thought to improve cardiovascular health and protect against heart attacks and strokes. This assumption is based on the belief that dietary saturated fat increases blood cholesterol, thus promoting cardiovascular disease. Total cholesterol has proven to have little correlation to heart disease and is a very poor indicator of risk. The reason for this is that total cholesterol includes HDL, the good cholesterol that protects against heart disease, and both large (good) and small (potentially bad) LDL, and you don't know how much of each makes up the total. This is why half of those people who suffer heart attacks have normal to even optimal total cholesterol levels. For this reason, doctors use different methods to evaluate risk. The cholesterol ratio (total cholesterol/HDL) is a far more accurate indicator of heart disease risk because it takes into account how much HDL makes up the total cholesterol.

Saturated fats tend to raise both HDL and large LDL cholesterol, both of which are beneficial. Thus, total cholesterol may rise. Sugar and refined starch tend to raise small LDL, the type that is easily oxidized and contributes to atherosclerosis and heart disease. Too much polyunsaturated vegetable oil tends to lower total cholesterol. It does this by reducing HDL and the good large LDL, with is not good.

Because our understanding of cholesterol and its role in the body has evolved over the years, there has been much debate over whether saturated fat actually promotes heart disease or not. Yes, some saturated fats do raise total cholesterol, but the vast majority of this is the good kind. It is sugar, refined starch, and processed vegetable oils that lower the good and raise the bad cholesterol. This coincides precisely with the history of coronary heart disease. Prior to the 1900s when animal fats dominated our diet, heart disease was rare. As these fats were replaced by vegetable and hydrogenated oils and as sugar and refined starch consumption increased in the 20th century, heart disease rates increased as well.

In order to resolve the debate, researchers from the Oakland Research Institute and Harvard School of Public Health conducted a study to analyze all of the available published studies with data for dietary saturated fat intake and risk of cardiovascular disease.

The studies also had to be of high quality and reliable. Twenty-one studies were identified that fit their criteria. This meta-analysis study included data on nearly 350,000 subjects. With such a large subject database, the results would be far more reliable than any of the individual studies with a much smaller number of subjects. The focus of the researchers was to determine if there was sufficient evidence linking saturated fat consumption to cardiovascular disease. Their results said "no." Intake of saturated fat was not associated with an increased risk of cardiovascular disease. Those people who ate the greatest amount of saturated fat were no more likely to suffer a heart attack or stroke than those who ate the least. It didn't matter how much saturated fat one ate, the incidence of heart disease was not affected. This study demonstrated that the combined data from all available studies in the medical literature disproves the idea that saturated fat promotes heart attacks and strokes.[6] A number of studies published more recently have confirmed these results; saturated fat does not cause heart disease. In fact, the studies indicate that sugar and refined starch intake is more closely linked to heart disease than fat is.[7-9]

5

Keto Cycling

THE MISSING LINK IN ANCESTRAL DIETS

It is reasoned that if we can get back to eating more like people had in the past when they consumed only whole, natural foods, and eliminate sugar and other highly processed foods, health would improve. Indeed, this is what happens. This is why ancestral diets have become so popular in recent years. People lose unwanted weight and feel much better. Often, even longstanding health problems such as arthritis or inflammatory bowel disease disappear.

However, there are those who do not see the remarkable improvements reported by others. They may lose a little weight, find their arthritis pain a little less painful, or have less digestive trouble, but the problems still persist. They follow the diet as they are instructed, so why aren't they feeling better than they do?

There is one very important element that has been a part of all ancestral diets from the beginning of time that is missing from nearly all modern versions of these diets. Adding this missing element can make any ancestral diet far more effective in preventing and reversing chronic and degenerative disease. This missing element is periodic fasting.

Our ancestors did not have access to the abundance of foods that we enjoy today. They didn't have the luxury of eating three meals a day. Often, they were lucky to get one meal daily. They had to search and hunt for their food. When the hunt wasn't successful, they went hungry. When crops failed or were devastated by droughts, insects, animals, and disease, they went hungry. Our ancestors missed a lot of meals and went for days, weeks, and sometimes even months with little to eat. Adding periodic or intermittent fasting to an ancestral diet can more accurately mimic the eating patterns of our ancestors and provide the missing element that can stop and even reverse chronic and degenerative disease—the so-called diseases of modern civilization.

It is the cycling between feast and famine that triggers survival mechanisms in our body that make it possible for us to overcome physical degeneration and regain our health.

STEM CELLS AND TISSUE REGENERATION

Our health and the health of our entire body depend on the health of our cells. All disease is cellular. The reason some people have kidney problems is because the cells in their kidneys are diseased or damaged; likewise, heart disease is caused by damaged heart (cardiac) cells. Any organ that contains damaged cells becomes less efficient and less functional. The more damaged or diseased the cells in an organ become, the more dysfunctional the organ. This is what leads to chronic disease.

The opposite is also true. The greater the number of healthy cells an organ contains, the better it functions. If all the cells in your kidneys were strong and healthy, your kidneys would function properly and efficiently. If all of the cells in your heart were healthy and resistant to disease, your heart would be healthy and resistant to disease. If all of the cells in your entire body were healthy and resistant to disease, what would that make you? It would make you healthy and resistant to disease! If our cells are healthy, so are we. If they are diseased and sick, so are we. Fortunately, there is a way to banish sick cells and replace them with newer, healthier cells, reverse chronic poor health, and slow down the aging process. The key to this remarkable process is the activation of stem cells—the type of cells that created our entire bodies.

Human cells, as they age, go through a progressive and irreversible series of changes until they reach a state at which they can no longer function properly and consequently die. Young stem cell-generated cells are plump, round, and smooth. As they age, they become irregular in shape, flatten out, enlarge, and fill up with debris; cell division slows down and eventually stops, which is ultimately followed by the death of the cell.

One of the signs of cellular aging is the increase in protein content of cells. This occurs as a result of incomplete division of the cell's contents during mitosis (cell division). Cells tend to accumulate residual debris—fragments of DNA—and often end up with multiple nuclei that have not properly separated. At some point, the cell is so littered with this debris and the DNA is so damaged that the cell

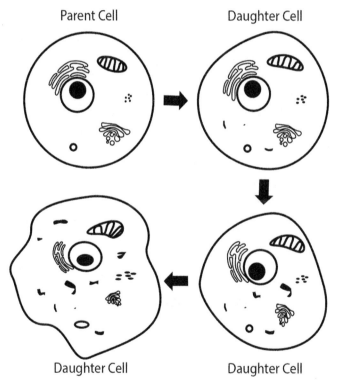

As you age, your cells and organelles (cell organs) undergo damage and mutations that affect how well they function. We are only as healthy as our cells. The more damaged cells in our bodies, the older we look and feel and the more prone we are to degenerative disease.

dies. However, up to that point the cell continues to multiply and divide, producing daughter cells. Daughter cells aren't like the cells produced from stem cells, which are the equivalent of newborn babies with a full lifetime ahead of them, but instead are copies of their parents, misshapen and filled with debris. In fact, the daughter cells tend to be in worse shape with more accumulative debris and more degeneration. This is why older cells and tissues become less functional with age. For example, old worn out pancreatic beta cells may no longer produce normal amounts of insulin, adrenal cells may no longer produce norepinephrine, ovaries may not produce estrogen, or the thyroid may no longer produce adequate amounts of thyroxine (T4). During autophagy, these older cells are removed, recycled, and eventually replaced by healthy new stem cell-generated cells.

The first cells to develop when an egg is fertilized are stem cells. These are not skin, bone, or liver cells, but undifferentiated cells that can transform into any type of cell through the activation of specific genes. During the first few days of life, the embryo consists completely of stem cells. These stem cells divide to form daughter stem cells, each containing an identical set of genes. As the embryo grows, certain genes are "turned on," causing the stem cells to transform into specialized cells that give rise to all the organs and tissues in the body.

After birth and throughout life, a few stem cells remain in the body to generate replacements for cells that are lost through normal wear and tear, injury, or disease. Once a stem cell has transformed into a specialized cell, it never reverts back to a stem cell, and its daughter cells are always of the same type. Once a stem cell becomes a bone or a brain cell, or any other type of cell, it remains that type of cell with an inherent limited life expectancy. Stem cells, however, can live indefinitely, giving rise to daughter stem cells. Since stem cells can become any type of cell in the body, they have the potential to regenerate any tissue or organ. Stem cells generally remain relatively dormant until genes are activated to trigger their transformation into specific types of cells.

Given the unique regenerative abilities of stem cells, scientists are currently developing ways to use them to treat certain diseases and injuries. The most important potential medical application of human stem cells is in the generation of cells and tissues for use in

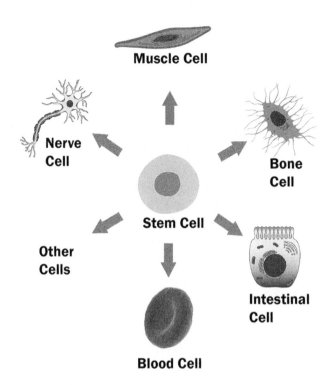

Muscle Cell

Nerve Cell

Bone Cell

Stem Cell

Other Cells

Intestinal Cell

Blood Cell

Stem cells can transform into any type of cell, replacing old damaged cells with new healthy cells.

cell-based therapies in which stem cells are induced to differentiate into the specific cell type required to repair damaged or destroyed cells or tissues. Currently, donated organs and tissues are often used to replace diseased or destroyed tissue, but the need for transplantable tissues and organs far outweighs the available supply. Stem cells, directed to differentiate into specific cell types, offer the possibility of a renewable source of replacement cells and tissues to treat diseases including macular degeneration, spinal cord injury, stroke, burns, heart disease, diabetes, osteoarthritis, and rheumatoid arthritis.

Cardiovascular disease, which includes hypertension, coronary heart disease, stroke, and congestive heart failure, can deprive heart tissue of oxygen, thereby killing cardiac muscle cells. This loss triggers a cascade of detrimental events, including the formation of scar tissue, an overload of blood flow and pressure capacity and the overstretching of viable cardiac cells attempting to sustain cardiac output. This in turn leads to heart failure and eventual death. Restoring damaged heart muscle tissue through repair or regeneration is therefore a promising new strategy to treat heart failure.

The use of stem cells for cardiac repair is an active area of research. A number of stem cell types, including embryonic stem cells, cardiac stem cells, myoblasts (muscle stem cells), adult bone marrow-derived cells, endothelial progenitor cells (cells that give rise to the endothelium, the interior lining of blood vessels), and umbilical cord blood cells, have been investigated as possible sources for regenerating damaged heart tissue. All have been explored in mouse or rat models, and some have been tested in larger animal models, such as pigs. A few small studies have also been carried out in humans, usually in patients who are undergoing open-heart surgery. Several of these have demonstrated that stem cells injected into the circulation or directly into the injured heart tissue appear to improve cardiac function and/or induce the formation of new capillaries. The mechanism for this repair remains controversial, and the stem cells likely regenerate heart tissue through several pathways. Although much more research is needed to assess the safety and improve the efficacy of this approach, these preliminary clinical experiments show how stem cells may one day be used to repair damaged heart tissue, thereby reversing cardiovascular disease.

In people who suffer from type 1 diabetes, the cells of the pancreas that normally produce insulin are destroyed by the patient's own immune system. Recent studies indicate that it may be possible to direct the differentiation of human stem cells in cell culture to form insulin-producing cells that eventually could be used in transplantation therapy for persons with diabetes.

To realize the potential of cell-based therapies for such pervasive and debilitating diseases, scientists must be able to manipulate stem cells so that they possess the necessary characteristics for successful differentiation, transplantation, and engraftment. In order to achieve this goal, scientists must learn to manipulate stem cells to reliably accomplish the following:

- Proliferate extensively and generate sufficient quantities of cells for making tissue.
- Differentiate into the desired cell type(s).

- Survive in the recipient after transplant.
- Integrate into the surrounding tissue after transplant.
- Function appropriately for the duration of the recipient's life.
- Avoid harming the recipient in any way.

Also, to avoid the problem of immune rejection, scientists are experimenting with different research strategies to generate tissues that will not be rejected.

As promising as stem cell therapy is, these are major challenges yet to be resolved. Fortunately, there is another option that does not require surgery, injections, tissue cultures, or risk of rejection, and does not cause any harm to the patient, does not require hospital or clinic visitation, and costs little. The alternative is a natural form of stem cell therapy instigated through fasting and keto cycling.

THE CLEANSING AND HEALING POWER OF AUTOPHAGY

One of the primary benefits of fasting is autophagy—the cannibalization of body tissues for recycling. As blood glucose declines during a fast, the body begins to cannibalize fat to fuel its energy needs. Most of the cells in our bodies do just fine using fatty acids and ketones as fuel; however, some cells absolutely require glucose. If you are fasting and not eating any sources of glucose, where does the glucose come from to feed these cells? It comes from protein. Where does this protein come from? It comes from you, from body tissues. Protein is broken down and converted into glucose in a process called gluconeogenesis. Our bodies have a keen sense of self preservation, so vital organs like your heart, liver, and kidneys are not touched. The first sources of protein the body cannibalizes are those that are of the least importance to your survival; this includes all old, worn out or dysfunctional cells and abnormal growths. The body essentially goes into housecleaning mode and cleans out fat and all of the cells and tissues that serve no useful function. It is only when fasting becomes prolonged that the body starts to dismantle more essential tissues like functional cells in our muscles and organs.

Most people would assume that during a fast, when we are depriving ourselves of food and nourishment, we would become weak and be vulnerable to disease. However, just the opposite happens, we become stronger and more resistant to disease.

Valter Longo, PhD and his team at the University of Southern California have been researching the effects of fasting on the immune system. He conducted an interesting study using mice that demonstrated how fasting can strengthen the body. He separated the mice into two groups. The first group was put on a 48-hour water fast. The second group served as the control and received their normal scientifically-designed, vitamin-fortified chow, supplying them with all the nutrients they needed to maintain optimal health. The mice in both groups were then injected with a lethal dose of poison. The poison chosen was a chemotherapy drug injected at an amount equivalent to about four times what a human cancer patient would receive. The mice receiving the nutritious diet immediately became deathly ill and lethargic; 65 percent of them died within a couple of days. The mice that were fasting, however, were running around as they normally do as if nothing happened. None of them died. The results were so shocking that Longo thought they may have done something wrong, so they repeated the experiment but ended up with the same outcome.

One thing that Longo and his team were not fully aware of at the time was the incredible power of ketones. Ketones not only act as an alternative source of energy to glucose, but trigger the activation of many survival mechanisms in the body, along with the upregulation of protective genes. When glucose is burned by the mitochondria in our cells to produce energy, destructive free radicals are created as a waste product from this process, much like gasoline burning in an automobile expels exhaust. The constant use of glucose as fuel puts a heavy strain on the antioxidant systems of the body. This can lead to depletion of our antioxidant reserves, allowing free radicals to run wild, breaking down our cells and tissues and promoting premature aging. Antioxidant nutrients such as vitamins A, C, D, and E can become quickly exhausted, leading to vitamin deficiencies. In other words, relying too much on glucose for energy can seriously lower your vitamin status and accelerate aging. An aging body is less effective in neutralizing and removing toxins, fighting off infections, and eliminating cancer and other damaged or dysfunctional cells. Ketones provide a much cleaner source of fuel—a superfuel in fact, because it produces more energy than glucose with far less pollution (free radicals). It is, in effect, a "green" fuel for the body. During ketosis, much fewer free radicals are produced, preserving antioxidant reserves and nutrient status and preventing much of the harm free radicals cause.

Ketones also calm inflammation, activate special proteins that help regulate homeostasis, trigger DNA repair, and aid in the detoxification process. Ketones improve the oxygen utilization of cells, making them more efficient and stronger. For example, during ketosis the hydraulic output of the heart muscle can improve substantially. Brain function also improves, which is one of the reasons why epileptic patients respond so dramatically to the ketogenic diet. Ketones have a remarkable ability to protect the body from the harmful effects of many toxins, including chemotherapy drugs.[1] This is why the drug administered to Longo's fasting mice had little to no effect and why the animals survived. After the fast, the immune system is strengthened with an increased ability to fight off infection and rogue cancer cells, providing further protection from harm.

Longo observed that during a fast, white blood cell numbers decline but as soon as refeeding begins, the white blood cell count quickly returns to normal. Studying the process more thoroughly, he discovered it was simply part of the process of autophagy. When fasting, the body removes all the old, worn out white blood cells (to be converted into glucose). He then observed that after a period of fasting, when food is reintroduced, stem cells in the bone marrow are activated and produce new white blood cells. Through this process, old, dysfunctional white blood cells are replaced with new, functional white blood cells. In essence, fasting generated a more robust and functional immune system.

The treatment for cancer using chemotherapy is accompanied by many awful side effects including, hair loss, fatigue, weakness, nausea, diarrhea, mouth sores, memory loss, and numbness—all a consequence of the toxic effects of the drugs. One of the main problems with chemo is that it destroys the immune system. It kills the white blood cells and the bone marrow where white blood cells are formed and has long lasting effects that make the patient vulnerable to infections and other health problems.

Longo found that fasting immediately before and after undergoing chemotherapy maintains proper immune function and eliminates the side effects of chemo, while also improving the effectiveness of the therapy. Fasting during chemotherapy has always been discouraged because it was believed to weaken the body, so cancer patients are always encouraged to eat more while undergoing this treatment. As Longo discovered, fasting doesn't weaken the body. Rather, it makes it stronger and protects the immune system from the damaging effects of chemo.

Longo reasoned that since fasting can regenerate the immune system, it might be useful in treating people suffering from immune disorders, particularly those with autoimmune diseases such as multiple sclerosis (MS), type 1 diabetes, rheumatoid arthritis, celiac disease, Hashimoto's thyroiditis, and lupus. Autoimmune diseases are believed to be caused by a dysfunctional immune system that attacks its own body.

Multiple sclerosis (MS) is a potentially disabling autoimmune disorder that affects the brain and spinal cord. The immune system attacks the nerve cells, destroying the protective myelin sheath that covers the nerve axon. This causes the cells to degenerate and disrupts communication between the brain and the rest of the body.

Drug therapy and dietary approaches to treating MS have been generally disappointing. For this reason, stem cell transplants are being investigated as a means to stop the progression of the disease. In this approach, the doctor uses the patients' own stem cells to reboot

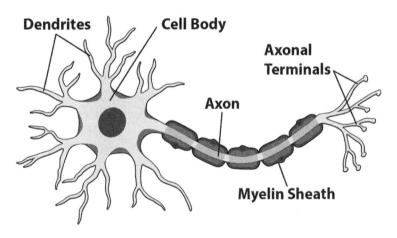

Nerve Cell

the immune system and stop the advance of the disease. Blood cells are formed from stem cells in the bone marrow. The treatment can be risky because after a specimen of bone marrow is removed, the patient's immune system has to be completely destroyed before the stem cells are transplanted back into the body. The treatment works best with younger patients with mild symptoms. So far, only half of the patients who have received this treatment see any benefit, with a nearly 3 percent fatality rate. This is of concern because MS itself is not life-threatening.[2]

Using stem cells to revitalize the immune system is a clever idea, but using stem cell transplants to accomplish this has not yet been too successful. A far safer and more effective approach is to use the body's own powers of immune system rejuvenation. Fasting can accomplish the same thing without the health risks.

"We started thinking," says Longo,"if [fasting] kills a lot of immune cells and turns on the stem cells, is it possible that maybe it will kill the bad ones and then generate new good ones?" The effect would be similar to that of a stem cell transplant, but without the risks. That inspired him to start investigating the effects of fasting on MS.

His study consisted of two parts. The first part used three groups of mice that had the equivalent of MS. The first group of mice cycled in and out of a 3-day fast three times over a 30-day period. The second group was put on a mild ketogenic diet. The third group served as the control and ate a normal diet. At the end of 30 days the mice in both the fasting and ketogenic groups were showing significant improvement. Analysis of nerve tissue showed that the myelin covering on the nerves were being regenerated. Going through the fasting cycle not only regenerated the animals' immune systems but also stimulated the regeneration of the damaged nerves. Through the process of autophagy dysfunctional white blood cells and damaged nerve cells were removed and replaced with new healthy cells. The mice in these two groups, and especially the fasting group, had improved so much that 20 percent of them had completely recovered from MS—quite a remarkable feat since there is no medical cure for this disease.

The second part of the study involved human subjects with MS. The participants were separated into three groups. The first group was put on a periodic fast separated by a high-fat Mediterranean type diet.

The second group was put on a ketogenic diet, and the third group ate a normal diet. After 6 months the first two groups of patients reported significant improvement in their MS symptoms. The third group showed no improvement. Again, the fasting and ketogenic diet proved beneficial.

Longo then examined the effects of fasting on another autoimmune disorder, type 1 diabetes. In this form of diabetes, the insulin producing beta cells in the pancreas are attacked and destroyed by the immune system, leading to diabetes. Mice with type 1 diabetes were used in this study. One group of mice was put on a four-day fasting cycle. Another group received their normal diet. The fasting mice had their immune systems regenerated. Old, dysfunctional white blood cells that had attacked the pancreas were replaced by new, healthy white blood cells. In addition, the damaged pancreatic beta cells were removed (recycled) and replaced with new, functional cells that produced insulin. These mice were now producing insulin with greatly improved blood sugar control. The fasting cycles switched on genes that activated pancreatic stem cells to form new insulin-producing beta cells. Again, Longo succeeded in reversing what was considered an irreversible condition.[3]

Longo and his team also studied the effects of fasting on mice with a genetic mutation that caused insulin resistance and type 2 diabetes. In the initial stages of this form of diabetes, a normal amount of insulin is produced, but if the condition is not well managed, the disease can damage pancreatic insulin-producing beta cells. In this case, supplemental insulin would be needed just as it is for type 1 diabetes. Mice used in this study had late-stage type 2 diabetes and thus could not produce insulin on their own. The mice were cycled on a 4 day fast, which resulted in the regeneration of insulin production in the pancreas and reversal of insulin resistance, allowing the animals to regain healthy blood glucose levels. Although this study was done on mice, the scientists also looked at the effects of fasting on human pancreatic cell cultures from diabetic donors and found that the cells responded in a similar manner.

In most of his animal and human studies, Longo didn't use a simple water fast but used what he calls a *fasting mimicking diet*—a diet that allows a limited amount of calories but mimics the metabolic and therapeutic effects of fasting. His fasting mimicking diet is a low-carb, low-protein, low-calorie, high-fat diet. It is basically a low-calorie ketogenic diet.

Longo's studies have shown that the fasting mimicking diet done in a series of short 4- or 5-day cycles can effectively reduce elevated levels of C-reactive protein (CRP), a marker for inflammation. CRP is elevated in many chronic diseases, including heart disease, diabetes, and inflammatory bowel diseases (IBD) like Crohn's disease and ulcerative colitis.

In a study published in the journal *Cell Reports*, Longo and colleagues demonstrated that cycling in and out of a fasting mimicking diet can effectively reduce systemic and intestinal inflammation in humans and mice and reverse the damage to the intestines caused by IBD.[4] The research team also observed activation of stem cells and a regenerative effect in the colon and the small intestine, which was evident only with multiple cycles of the fasting mimicking diet. They concluded that fasting primes the body for improvement, but it is the refeeding that provides the opportunity to rebuild cells and tissues. "It is really remarkable, that in the past 100 years of research into calorie restriction, no one recognized the importance of the refeeding." Longo says. Cycling through the diet not only calmed inflammation and stimulated the removal and replacement of damaged tissue, but promoted the growth of beneficial gut microorganisms.

One of the advantages of the fasting mimicking diet over a juice or water fast is that it includes the health-promoting fiber from the vegetables and nuts included in the diet, which support a healthy gut microbiome. Longo has found that the very low-calorie diet produces better results than a water only fast. In this study, two cycles of a 4-day fasting mimicking diet followed by a normal diet was enough to mitigate inflammatory bowel disease-associated symptoms. In comparison, a water-only fast came up short, indicating that certain nutrients in the fasting mimicking diet contributed to the microbial and anti-inflammatory changes necessary to maximize the effects of the diet. "We've determined that the dietary components are contributing to the beneficial effects; it's not just about the cells of the human body but it's also about the microbes that are affected by both the fasting and the diet." Longo said. "The ingredients in the diet pushed the microbes to help the fasting maximize the benefits against inflammatory bowel disease."

Longo recommends a fasting mimicking diet for individuals who want to take advantage of the health benefits of fasting without the discomfort of going completely without eating. On his program, total calorie intake is limited to about 800 calories a day for a total of 5 consecutive days. He recommends doing the diet once a month for optimal benefit. It is important to go in and out of the fast to allow the body to go through the complete cleansing and rebuilding cycle.

It must be emphasized that in order for this diet to have the greatest therapeutic effect, both carbohydrate and protein must be restricted. Carbohydrate must be limited in order to shift the body into ketosis so that it burns primarily fat. Protein must be restricted to activate housecleaning, initiate the cannibalization of worn out cells and tissues, and revive the immune system. Limiting carbohydrate intake stimulates the breakdown of fat. Limiting protein intake stimulates the breakdown of protein—old, dysfunctional tissue. The fasting mimicking diet consists primarily of low-carb vegetables and fat.

THE FEASTING-FASTING CYCLE

Many people wanting to lose excess weight or achieve better health have found the ketogenic diet to be the most effective means they have ever tried. Some people have had limited success with other diets, but the problem is that when they go off their diet, the weight and poor health gradually return. The ketogenic diet has many advantages over these other diets. It allows you to eat a variety of delicious, satisfying foods that are forbidden on low-fat diets, and you can eat until satisfied without starving yourself. The foods are nutrient dense, so they provide complete nutrition to support good health. Unlike a low-fat, calorie-restricted diet that over the long-term promotes malnutrition, the ketogenic diet can be maintained indefinitely.

For this reason, some people believe that they should stay on the ketogenic diet for extended periods of time, even for life. As good as the ketogenic diet is, it is best not to remain on the diet continually or for long periods of time.

Ketosis is the term used to indicate when the body is using fat and ketones as its primary source of fuel. In contrast, I use the term *glucosis* to describe the metabolic state when the body is using glucose as its primary source of fuel. When we are fasting or eating a ketogenic diet, we go into ketosis. When we are eating a normal diet that includes carbohydrates, we are in glucosis. Most people spend almost all of their lives in glucosis.

The ketogenic diet was developed to mimic the metabolic and therapeutic effects of fasting. Like fasting, it shifts the body into ketosis, using fat as the primary source of fuel. Blood glucose and insulin levels are maintained at low, but normal, healthy levels. Certain genes and processes are upregulated or switched on and others are downregulated or switched off. The body shifts into a state of intense housecleaning or catabolism wherein fat and dysfunctional proteins are broken down and removed. You do not want to remain in state of cleansing or catabolism continually. It can be beneficial for a time, but not perpetually. You also need a period of time for rebuilding. When refeeding resumes the body receives an influx of energy and nutrients that triggers rebuilding, repair, and growth.

Shifting from glucosis to ketosis is like turning on a switch that activates autophagy and internal housecleaning. Shifting from ketosis to glucosis turns on the switch that promotes rebuilding and repair. Every time we shift from one state to another we activate processes that improve our health. For this reason, it is to our advantage to cycle between glucosis and ketosis on a regular basis.

Fasting is much like exercising a muscle. Exercise causes the breakdown of tissue, but resting afterwards allows these tissues to rebuild and become stronger and healthier. It is during the rest period that the muscles actually grow and you benefit from the exercise. It is much the same with ketosis. When you start to eat again it stimulates growth, repair, and healing. Fasting breaks things down, refeeding builds them back up stronger and healthier. Staying in ketosis long-term doesn't allow for these benefits to occur, just as over exercising doesn't allow the muscles to recuperate and strengthen. Switching from fat burning to sugar burning activates genes and triggers the generation of stem cells. When you stay in either state long-term, old dysfunctional cells divide and multiply, producing more dysfunctional daughter cells. When you switch from fat burning to sugar burning, you activate stem cells to produce completely new functional cells to replace the old dysfunctional ones. This is exactly what Valter Longo found in his fasting studies.

Even though you may initially see benefits, staying too long in ketosis can become counterproductive. When you stay in ketosis for an extended period of time, your body begins to adapt to the elevated level of ketones and the therapeutic effects begin to decline. Just as continually eating a high-carb diet can condition the body so that it does not metabolize fat efficiently, a ketogenic diet can condition the body so that it does not metabolize carbohydrate efficiently. Long-term keto can make you more sensitive to the starch and sugar in your diet, elevating blood glucose levels. This is one of the reasons why when traditional meat eating populations such as the Inuit and American Plains Indians were established on permanent settlements and given sugar, white flour, and other high-carbohydrate foods, they quickly developed diabetes.

Cycling in and out of ketosis keeps the body primed to easily and quickly switch to burning either fat or sugar, allowing ketones to maintain their full therapeutic power. A healthy diet is also important both when you are on and off the ketogenic diet.

When our ancestors went without food or only had access to a little food, they naturally went into a state of nutritional ketosis. They were cycling in and out of ketosis constantly throughout the year and throughout their lives. This keto cycling, combined with a healthy traditional diet, protected them from chronic degenerative disease. Of course, if the period of fasting or severe food depravation lasted too long it could lead to starvation, but as long as the periods of fasting were limited to just a few days to a few weeks at a time and were separated by periods of relative abundance, the people thrived and were healthy. Cycling in and out of ketosis is completely natural and highly beneficial.

A UNIVERSAL LAW OF NATURE

Cycling is a universal of law of nature. Everything in nature goes through cycles, even the earth itself. The earth and planets move in set patterns which create the cycle of day and night, the ebb and flow of the tides, the turning of the seasons, and the forces that shape climate patterns.

The cycle of life follows a well defined pattern. Single-celled microorganisms feed on bacteria. These microorganisms are, in turn, eaten by tiny multicellular organisms, which are consumed by larger animals, who in turn are eaten by larger animals on up through the food chain to the apex consumer. The animal at the top of the food chain eventually dies and is consumed by the tiniest of all the bacteria, and the cycle repeats itself.

The natural environment follows a cycle. For example, forests can be destroyed by a lightning strike that causes a fire leaving the ground bare. Grasses move in to dominate the landscape, followed by larger scrubs, and then finally trees, each set of plants accompanied by its unique insect and animal life. In time the forest returns, only to be devastated again by fire, which allows the cycle to repeat itself.

The earth and its crust go through cycles in which rocks are created and destroyed and then created again. Molten rock cools to form mountains of hardened lava and granite. These rocks are weathered and are gradually broken down into boulders, gravel, sand, silt, and clay. Through the action of heat, pressure, and chemical changes, they are reformed into new rock—sedimentary and metamorphic rocks— or are reabsorbed into the earth at subduction zones and turned back into molten rock to begin the process all over again.

Throughout history the life on this planet has existed in a cyclical environment with periods of time when food was abundant and times when it wasn't. This is the environment that predominated throughout all of human history until just recently. The earth cycles through phases of feast and famine as it cycles through each of the seasons. Spring and summer is a time of growth and renewal while fall and winter is when growth stops and much of the life on the planet dies or goes into a state of dormancy. Each cycle brings on a renewal in life. As winter ends and spring begins, new shoots emerge from the ground. Trees and shrubs awake from dormancy and sprout blossoms and leaves. Animals give birth. Life springs up everywhere. Even on a day to day basis we see a cycle of dormancy (night) and activity (day). It is like hitting a reset button, the time of dormancy, decay, and breaking down is replaced with new growth and activity.

Eating in cycles between feasting and fasting is part of the natural order of nature. It is the pattern in which all wildlife has existed from the beginning of time. Animals removed from their natural cycle to live as pets often get fat and sick just like us and develop human degenerative diseases like arthritis, cancer, diabetes, kidney and liver disease, high blood pressure, and such. Veterinarians report that nearly half of our dogs are overweight or obese, just as we are. It has gotten so bad that you can even buy health insurance for your pets to reduce the costs of expensive medication and veterinary treatment. Eating too much and too often is the underlying cause for these conditions. In the wild, where animals live as nature intended, they do not experience these health problems and do not need health insurance.

Our health is directly connected to nature's cycles, and healers throughout the ages have noted this. Our bodies are designed to follow the natural cycle of eating with the seasons and experiencing periods of feast and famine. Old-time doctors experienced in treating patients using fasting therapy found that multiple periods of fasting are generally necessary in order to successfully treat patients with serious chronic disease. Fasting multiple times (cycling) is generally more effective than doing just one very long fast.

Dr. John R. Christopher (1909-1983), was one of America's most renowned herbalists and founded the School of Natural Health, an organization that has trained thousands of herbalists. He taught the principle of cycling when treating patients with herbal remedies. If the treatment required many weeks, he put his patients on a 7-day cycle that involved taking the herbal treatment for 6 days, followed by a 1 day rest. He found that by doing this his patients responded more quickly to the treatment. He noticed that treatments tended to lose their efficiency when applied repeatedly every single day over an extended period of time. Cycling in and out of treatment by giving the patient a short rest prevented the body from developing resistance or adapting to the treatment.

The same can happen in drug therapy as well. Patients often see a decline in the effectiveness of a drug they are using, and their doctors have to prescribe a different drug to get the desired results. Pain medications, especially addictive drugs, often have a similar effect. At first, they work really well, but over time the body adapts to the medication and the drugs become less effective. At this point, a stronger dose is needed to get the same results.

Our health improves when we follow the cycle of nature and go through periods of feast and famine. It is contrary to natural law for us to be continually eating, consuming three full meals a day plus snacks. It is this overindulgence in food that has led to most of our chronic health problems today.

A LIFESTYLE CHANGE

Keto cycling makes it possible to adopt a dietary change that is doable for a lifetime. Low-fat, calorie-restricted diets almost always fail over time because they are viewed as temporary measures to lose a certain amount of weight or achieve some goal. Once the goal has been achieved or you become sick and tired of dieting, you go back to eating the way you used to—the way that made you fat and sick in the first place. Before long, you have regained the weight you lost and your health has declined. You are right back where you started.

In order to make a permanent change in your health, the diet chosen must be part of a lifestyle change. The diet must be one that could be maintained for life. Most weight loss diets are not suitable for a lifetime because they are too restrictive, unsatisfying, unpalatable, and generally unhealthy.

Many people try a ketogenic diet for a few weeks or months and then, like any weight loss diet, go back to eating the poor quality foods they were eating before. If you approach the ketogenic diet like any other diet, as a temporary means to an end, your long-term results will likely be no different.

In order to make the ketogenic diet powerful enough to achieve optimal health for life, the diet must be a part of a lifestyle change. Keto cycling makes this possible. When you cycle in and out of ketosis, you do not have to permanently give up all of the higher carb foods you love and can't live without. You simply refrain from eating them for the periods of time you are actively in ketosis. This way you don't feel deprived and temptation is not as intense. However, you should always avoid eating junk foods, both when you are in and out of ketosis. Low-carb junk foods should be avoided as well; simply because they are low-carb or even "keto" does not make them healthy. Your ketogenic diet and normal diet should be based on nutritious, whole, natural foods. This doesn't mean you can't enjoy a slice of birthday cake on occasion. In fact, keto cycling allows you this privilege. You can plan your cycles so that you are on your normal diet when special occasions, like birthdays and anniversaries, come around. That way you can have a treat without guilt and without it throwing you out of ketosis.

THE 12-DAY KETO CYCLE

Normally it takes between 3 to 7 days eating a ketogenic diet to get into a moderate state of ketosis. As your body adapts to going in and out of ketosis, you will be able to go into ketosis more quickly. Fasting the first 2 to 3 days is the quickest way to get into ketosis, but the first few days of fasting are always the most arduous. This is the time when hunger and temptation are the most intense and the primary reason why people find it difficult to fast and often fail. The ketogenic diet essentially eliminates this problem.

The ketogenic diet allows you to get into ketosis while eating full meals that completely satisfy your hunger. Once you are in ketosis, hunger substantially declines and skipping a meal or two doesn't seem difficult at all.

While the ketogenic diet will get you into ketosis, restricting your calorie intake will get you into a deeper level and enhance the health-promoting effects. Optimally, the ketogenic diet should include periods of fasting or semi-fasting, followed by a period of refeeding or feasting. I have found that the easiest and most effective way to do this is to start with a 7-day ketogenic diet followed by a 5-day fasting mimicking diet—a 12-day cycle. The first 3 to 4 days on the ketogenic diet you transition from glucosis to ketosis. This is the time when you will feel hunger as you normally do, so eat three meals if you need to and eat until satisfied. As you get more into ketosis your hunger will subside. In the next 3 to 4 days of the ketogenic diet phase, your hunger will be substantially depressed which will allow you to cut back on the amount of food you eat without too much difficulty. Here is where intermittent fasting becomes beneficial. Choose any method of intermittent fasting you like—I find the time-restricted fast to be well suited for this and easy to incorporate in the keto cycle. Limit the period in which you eat to 8 consecutive hours. You can choose any time of day that fits your schedule best. I like to begin eating breakfast after 9:00 am and finish dinner no later than 5:00 pm. This provides me with a period of 16 hours when I am fasting. Of course, the exact time can change according to circumstances. You can intensify the

The Keto Cycle

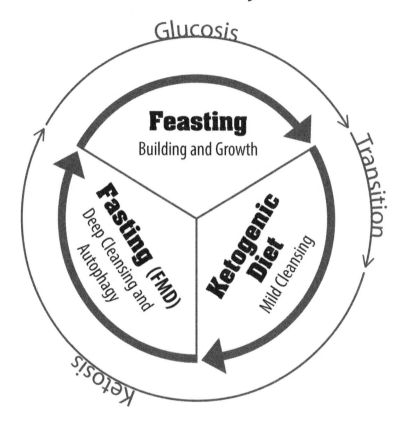

When food is eaten freely, the body is in a state of glucosis, using glucose as its primary source of fuel. This is the growth and building phase of the cycle. As a ketogenic diet is adopted there is a short transition period of a few days as the body switches from glucosis to ketosis and begins using fat as its primary source of fuel. Here the body enters a state of breaking down and cleansing. Moving into the fasting phase intensifies the body's reliance on fat for fuel and the processes of cleansing and autophagy. The cycle repeats as eating is resumed.

fast by extending the fasting period to 18 or 20 hours and shortening the feeding time to 6 or 4 hours, respectively.

After 7 days on the ketogenic diet (and intermittent fasting), the next 5 days should consist of a series of 24-hour fasts—fasting from dinner one day to dinner the next. Here is an excellent opportunity to do a very low-calorie, low-carb, low-protein, moderate-fat diet—essentially a fasting mimicking diet. Limit your total daily calories to 600 or less; 200 to 300 of these calories should come from healthy fats such as coconut or olive oils. A tablespoon of oil contains 126 calories, so this would amount to about 2 to 3 tablespoons of oil. The remaining calories should come from low-carb vegetables and perhaps a small amount of low-carb nuts. It is very important that you do not include any high-protein foods such as meat, eggs, or cheese because you want to stimulate autophagy and do a thorough 5-day cleanse, just as if you were on a water fast.

After 5 days on the fasting mimicking diet, your cleansing state is over and you can begin eating a normal, healthy mixed diet. This is your feasting period in which your body shifts to rebuilding. You should increase your intake of healthy carbohydrates, which may include fruits, tubers, legumes, and perhaps even some whole grains. The total time you spend in ketosis (ketogenic diet, intermittent fasting, and fasting mimicking diet) is 12 days followed by a period of normal but healthy eating. The period of normal eating can last as long as you like—a week, 2 weeks, a month, or more. The important thing is to repeat the cycle multiple times throughout the year. You can run through the cycle every month or every other month, whatever works best for you.

In summary, the 12-day keto cycle consists of 7 days on a ketogenic diet, of which at least 3 to 4 days will also include intermittent fasting, generally a 16/8 or 18/6 pattern. The second phase consists of 5 days of fasting using the fasting mimicking diet. The third phase is refeeding and eating a normal, but healthy, diet. The refeeding time varies, but the time you are getting into and then remaining in ketosis is 12 days.

The fasting mimicking diet as described here is essentially a very low-calorie daily time-restricted intermittent fasting diet, in which the period of fasting is extended to nearly 24 hours and the window for eating is limited to about 20 minutes or so. Eating only one meal, especially a very low-calorie meal, can be difficult for some people. If you find it too hard to go without eating for 24 hours, you can ease up a little with the 20/4 hour version, fasting 20 hours and eating during the 4 hour window. If you do this, you should still limit total daily calorie intake to about 600 calories.

Keep in mind that it is when you are fasting that deep cleansing and autophagy are really effective and produce the best results. However, any level of fasting is beneficial, so don't get discouraged if you can't hold out for 20 or 24 hours or can't limit your food intake to 600 calories. Just do the best you can. Over time, you will become more accustomed to fasting and it will get easier to reach the 24 hour, 600 calorie goal.

You will find recipes for the fasting mimicking diet in Chapter 9.

VARIABLE-DAY CYCLES

You can extend the keto diet and/or fasting days into a 20-day or 30-day cycle if you like. It is highly beneficial to always end the cycle with at least a 5-day fasting mimicking diet. However, with longer cycle periods the fasting mimicking diet could extend to 7 or 10 days if desired. It is a good idea to do an extended cycle at least once a year to get in some deep cleansing that takes longer than 12 days. When water fasting, it has been observed that extended fasts of 20 to 30 days or more can accomplish positive results for some stubborn health problems that are difficult to resolve with shorter fasts. The same is true for keto cycling. Consider adding in a few water fasting or intermittent fasting days into your schedule. Our ancestors didn't have a schedule they followed. Rather, they went without or with little food randomlyfor periods of time that would last anywhere from a few days to several weeks.

I like to follow what was natural for our ancient ancestors. I do one long keto cycle each year during the winter when food was traditionally the scarcest. This cycle generally lasts about 6 to 8 weeks. In addition, I go on a 12 to 14 day cycle in early spring and again in the fall. I also do a 6:1 diet, where I do a full 24 hour water fast one day every week, 52 weeks of the year. Most days, whether I'm in keto or not, I follow a 16/8 eating pattern, fasting 16 hours and eating within a 8 hour window. I am approaching 70 years of age and my fasting blood sugar, A1C, insulin, CRP (inflammation), and other health markers are all within a healthy normal range and I take no medications. If I was battling a major health problem such as diabetes or atherosclerosis, I would be more aggressive and do the 12-day or a 20- or even 26-day keto cycle at least every month until my health improved. However, I've been doing periodic fasting and ketogenic dieting for many years.

People with very serious health issues, such as cancer, epilepsy, Alzheimer's, Parkinson's, and autism, need to be on a near continuous keto diet. They can benefit from a 29-day keto cycle done monthly. This means that they would be in the feasting stage for only 1 or 2 days per month. During this time, calorie intake can increase. Too many carbs, however, can have an adverse effect, so total carbohydrate intake should still be limited to about 100 to 150 grams/day during the feasting stage; this is still more than two to three times as much as an ordinary ketogenic diet. The carbohydrates consumed need to be healthy, rich in fiber, and low in sugar and be consumed with good sources of fat and protein so that glucose absorption into the bloodstream is slow and steady. Sweets and refined grains need to be avoided entirely.

6

The Healing Process

SYMPTOMS ASSOCIATED WITH KETOSIS

If you have been eating like most people do nowadays, you probably eat a lot of packaged, processed, and convenience foods. When you start doing the ketogenic diet you will notice some distinct changes in your health. Be prepared to feel good, bad, and sick. That's right. Sick. Before you get better, you may get worse—but only temporarily.

Ultimately you will be healthier than you have ever been in your life and feel great both physically and mentally. Mental and physical capacity will improve, energy will increase, and you will be happier and more positive about yourself and about life. You will lose unwanted weight, improve blood circulation, and look healthier. But before you reach this stage, you may experience some physical and psychological changes that might seem unpleasant.

As good as the ketogenic diet is for weight loss and general improvement in health, there are some people who cannot fathom the idea that a high-fat diet can be healthful and are quick to criticize it at every opportunity. As justification for their belief, they reel off a list of side effects that they have heard are often associated with the ketogenic diet such as a lack of energy, weakness, bad breath, diarrhea, constipation, headaches, muscle cramps, insomnia, and flu-like symptoms. Critics make it sound like everyone who tries a ketogenic diet will suffer from all or most of these disturbing conditions, which will plague them the entire time they are on the diet. Anyone who would willingly go on such a diet would have to be crazy.

Those who go on a ketogenic diet may experience some of these symptoms, but for the most part, all these side effects are temporary. Probably the most pronounced symptoms associated with the ketogenic diet are the initial feelings of fatigue and a decrease in exercise performance. When you first start the ketogenic diet, your body must switch from burning glucose as its primary source of fuel to burning fat. It takes time to make this transition. During this time you will feel a lack of energy and you may not perform physical activities as well as you normally did. Once your body has shifted to burning fat, you will be in nutritional ketosis. Energy levels will increase and your former endurance and exercise capacity will return. In fact, they both may improve.

When someone first goes on the ketogenic diet, energy and endurance will decline for two to three weeks before recovering. As you go in and out of ketosis multiple times, the body becomes more efficient at switching between sugar burning and fat burning and the transition time shortens. You will go into ketosis faster, and your energy levels will decline for only a few days.

The ketogenic diet is vastly different from the standard diet we normally eat. The consumption of carbohydrate, especially sugar and refined starch, is dramatically reduced. Sugar and even starch, which is nothing more than glucose, are highly addictive. Studies have shown that they are just as addictive as cocaine. In animal studies, sugar was shown to be even more addictive than cocaine. Rats offered both sugar and cocaine preferred the sugar. Even rats that were already addicted to cocaine quickly switched their addiction to sugar when given the choice between the two.[1] Most people don't realize how addictive sugar really is and don't recognize that they are addicted. Sugar is in so many foods that an addiction can be fueled by eating a variety of foods, not just obvious sugar-laden treats like ice cream and chocolate. When all of these high-sugar and high-starch foods are discontinued, it can lead to withdrawal symptoms. Besides cravings or desires for these foods, the most common symptom is headaches. After a few days in ketosis, the headaches will go away.

Addictions to caffeine, chocolate, bread (starch), drugs, and other substances will also be overcome if these items are avoided during the diet. Consequently, you may experience withdrawal symptoms like anxiety, cravings, and fatigue as well for a few days as the body fights to overcome the addiction.

The change in diet will also affect your digestive system. On the ketogenic diet, especially if you are also doing intermittent fasting, you will generally feel less hungry and consume less food. This reduction in food will be noticed as a reduction and frequency in bowel movements. Some people interpret this as constipation. It is not constipation, but instead just the natural consequence of eating less and thus producing less waste.

The ketogenic diet may also decrease your feelings of thirst, causing you to drink less often. This can lead to mild dehydration, which in turn can lead to constipation. The solution is to drink more water throughout the day. I recommend about six glasses daily.

Muscle cramps are an often reported side effect of ketosis. When in ketosis, many electrolytes are lost in perspiration, urine, and elsewhere. A deficiency in the important minerals magnesium, potassium, and sodium can lead to muscle cramps. For this reason, it is recommended that you include a mineral supplement in your diet. Sodium can be supplied by eating an ample amount of salt with your foods. If you feel constipated, magnesium will help move things along in a smooth manner to avoid that issue.

Some people complain that being in ketosis disturbs their sleep patterns and even causes insomnia. What is really happening is that the brain is functioning at a higher level of awareness and efficiency. Ketones provide more energy than glucose and the brain functions more effectively burning ketones. As a consequence, your brain becomes more alert and better able to focus and concentrate; you will also experience less drowsiness during the day. At night when your normal bedtime comes around, instead of being mentally fatigued, your mind will be alert. Some people interpret this as insomnia, but it is not. If you go to bed at your normal time, even if you don't feel drowsy like you normally would, you will still fall asleep just as quickly. If you wake up in the middle of the night, instead of feeling like you are in a sleepy haze, your mind will be immediately alert. If you just relax and clear your mind, you will quickly fall back to sleep and get a full night's rest. If you follow this pattern you will generally get a better night's sleep than you normally do. In the morning you will wake refreshed with more energy and alertness. Over time, you will become accustomed to this increased mental clarity and it will become natural and less noticeable.

Another very common symptom is bad breath. This is often mistakenly referred to as "keto breath." True keto breath has a sweet fruity smell and is *not* unpleasant. It is caused by the release of ketones in the breath. The bad breath that most people complain about when doing keto is a result of internal cleansing and detoxification. The smell comes not from ketones, but from putrid toxins that are being expelled from the body. Bad breath is usually accompanied by a white or yellow coated tongue, a clear sign of detoxification.

Some people report that being in ketosis can cause an upset stomach, aches, pains, sinus discharge, and feelings of general discomfort. These symptoms have been referred to as the "keto flu." This so-called keto flu, along with some of the other symptoms associated with ketosis such as bad breath, fatigue, headaches, and diarrhea, are all the result of the cleansing process. These symptoms are not unique to the ketogenic diet, as they are also associated with fasting and semi-fasting dieting (less than about 600 calories/ day) and are a result of the body's shift into autophagy and intense housecleaning.

DETOXIFICATION AND CLEANSING
A Sea of Toxins

We live in an environment teaming with toxins, both natural and manmade, that attack our bodies daily. We are exposed to potentially harmful toxins in the food we eat, the water we drink, the air we breathe, and the environment in which we live. Exposure to toxins in our daily life is unavoidable.

The amount of toxins in the world today is far greater than in generations past. Since the end of World War II, the world has been flooded with tens of thousands of manmade chemicals. Today, over 80,000 different chemicals are in common use, and many of them are highly toxic. Each year an estimated 5 billion pounds of chemical pollutants are released into our environment, and the amount is increasing every year.

Toxins are harmful substances that can alter your DNA and disrupt cellular function. They can modify gene expression, interfere with enzyme function, damage cell membranes, and disrupt hormone balance.

Our bodies are like sponges that soak up these toxins. Most of them are quickly intercepted by our immune system and flushed out of the body. However, many get incorporated into our cells and tissues, where they can remain for decades and even for life. Over time, our body accumulates more and more of this poisonous material, which adversely affects our health and promotes disease.

Roundup is the most commonly used pesticide used throughout the world. It is used on commercial crops as well as around homes and businesses. Roundup residue is common on all types of produce and even in meats. According to the FDA, Roundup has been found in virtually all foods they have tested, including crackers, orange juice, wine, ice cream, and honey. Glyphosate, the active ingredient in Roundup, has been detected in the bodies of 70 percent of people tested.[2] This is worrisome because glyphosate has been linked to an increased risk of cancer and fatty liver disease.

Glyphosate is just one of thousands of chemicals we are exposed to. If measurable levels are found in 70 percent of the population, how many other chemicals can be detected in the human body? A recent study by the US Center for Disease Control and Prevention (CDC) tested 2,400 people age 6 and older for 148 toxic compounds in their urine and blood. They found that most Americans are carrying dozens of pesticides and toxic chemicals that are used in consumer products in their bodies, including pyrethroids, which are in virtually every household pesticide, and phthalates, which are found in nail polish and other beauty products as well as soft plastics.[3] According to the nonprofit organization Environmental Working Group, the average newborn baby has 287 known toxins in his or her umbilical cord blood. If a newborn is exposed to that many toxins, imagine how many can be found in adults.

David Duncan, a journalist with *National Geographic* magazine, wanted to find out what substances build up inside the body of a typical American over a lifetime. He had himself tested for 320 chemicals and pollutants such as DDT and PCBs, lead, mercury, pesticides, and compounds found in shampoos, nonstick cookware, and fabrics. These tests are too expensive for most people, about $15,000. Fortunately, *National Geographic* paid the bill and had him report the results.[4]

Duncan's test showed the presence of trace amounts of several chemicals that have long been banned or restricted, including DDT and other pesticides such as the termite-killers chlordane and heptachlor; lead and dioxins, probably from contaminated water; and PCBs, used as electrical insulators and heat-exchange fluids in transformers and other products. PCBs can persist in the environment for decades. In animals, they impair liver function, raise blood lipids, and cause cancers. Some of the 209 different PCBs chemically resemble dioxins and cause other mischief in lab animals, such as reproductive and nervous system damage as well as developmental problems. Despite the fact that most of these toxins have not been used in the US for many years (for instance, DDT was banned in the United States in 1972) his body still contained the pesticide. DDT was banned for agricultural uses worldwide by 2001, but is still permitted in small quantities in some countries for special purposes.

Almost all of us collect phthalates, which are found in shampoo to dissolve fragrances, thicken lotions, and add flexibility to PVC, vinyl, and some plastic food wrap. Car dashboards are loaded with phthalates. Phthalates disrupt reproductive development in mice. Duncan's phthalate levels were unusually high, in the top 5 percent. The toxicologist working with him speculated that the high levels in Duncan's blood may have been due to him taking urine sample in the morning, just after he had showered and washed his hair. It is interesting that a single washing can absorb so much of this chemical.

Duncan's load of household chemicals included perfluorinated acids (PFAs)—tough, chemically resistant compounds that go into making nonstick and stain-resistant coatings. In animals these substances damage the liver, affect thyroid hormones, and cause birth defects and perhaps cancer. Duncan routinely used nonstick cookware.

Also found were several dioxins, which are highly toxic compounds produced as a byproduct in some manufacturing processes, notably herbicide production and paper bleaching. They are a serious and persistent environmental pollutant that settle on soil and in the water and then pass into the food chain. They build up in animal fat, and most people accumulate them from eating meat and dairy products.

There was also mercury, a neurotoxin that can permanently impair brain function. Coal-burning power plants have been a major source of mercury, sending it out their stacks into the atmosphere. In the environment, bacteria transform it into a form called methylmercury, which moves up the food chain after plankton absorb it from the water and are eaten by small fish. Large predatory fish at the top of the marine food chain, like tuna and swordfish, accumulate the highest concentrations of methylmercury and pass it on to seafood lovers.

The most worrisome toxins found in the tests were high levels of flame-retarding compounds called polybrominated diphenyl ethers (PBDE). In mice and rats, flame retardants at doses comparable to those found in Duncan interfere with thyroid function, cause reproductive and neurological problems, and affect learning, memory and behavior. They are used on fabrics and plastics to prevent fires from starting or to slow their speed. They are used on clothes, sheets, towels, carpets, drapes, upholstery, and other fabrics. Since they were introduced about 30 years ago, our world has become saturated with these chemicals. Flame retardants have been found throughout the world, including in polar bears in the Arctic and killer whales in the Pacific. They are often even present in human breast milk. Flame retardants escape from treated plastic and fabrics in dust particles or as gases that cling to dust. People inhale the dust. Infants crawling on the floor get an especially high dose.

Duncan was asked if he had recently bought new furniture or rugs, spends a lot time around computer monitors, or lives near a factory making flame retardants. He answered no to all of these questions. Did he travel a lot on airplanes? Yes, almost 200,000 miles (320,000 km) the previous year. Airplane plastic and fabric interiors are drenched in flame retardants to meet safety standards set by the Federal Aviation Administration and its counterparts in Europe and Asia.

Like Duncan, we too, have collected a lifetime of toxins in our bodies. In addition to industrial toxins, we also collect natural or biological toxins from microorganisms, plants, soil, toxic metals, and even metabolic waste. These toxins can remain with us for life unless we do something to purge them from the body. Fasting has proven to be the most effective method to accomplish this. The natural cleansing and detoxification action initiated by a fast flushes these toxins from our bodies. The ketogenic diet appears to do the same.

The Body's Power to Heal

Our bodies have an amazing capacity to heal themselves. We get a cut, break a bone, tear a muscle, or get an infection, and the body immediately goes to work to repair the damage and fix the problem. The body knows exactly what to do in every case—no matter how old it is, it never forgets how to repair itself. Like an army on constant patrol, our immune system silently defends us against the thousands of enemy attacks mounted against us every day. If the body is healthy, it can quickly heal injury and ward off countless diseases.

The immune system, liver, and kidneys are able to filter out and remove most of the toxins we are exposed to every day. What they can't eliminate immediately often collects in tissues, especially fatty tissue like our fat cells. The fatter you are, the more toxins you are likely to be holding. Fasting is a natural process that flushes these toxins out of the body.

During a fast, fat and protein in our bodies are broken down to produce energy. In the process, stored toxins are removed and released into the bloodstream. This huge influx of poisons can be very harmful and perhaps even deadly. The body is intelligent. It doesn't do things to kill itself. It has a superb means by which these toxins are rendered harmless and flushed out of the body. During a fast, as the body goes through autophagy and cleansing, it also produces ketones.

Ketones are a natural defense against harmful toxins in our environment and in our bodies. They are the most powerful broad-spectrum anti-toxin or detoxifying agents known. They can neutralize or weaken the effects a wide variety of potentially harmful substances including bacterial endotoxins and exotoxins, fungal mycotoxins, drugs, environmental pollutants, cellular waste, agricultural poisons and pesticides, carcinogens, chemical food additives (MSG, dyes, preservatives, etc.), and many assorted manmade chemicals. Ketones have been shown to be effective in neutralizing the harmful effects of dozens of natural and synthetic toxins.[5]

Dr. Valter Longo discovered the anti-toxin power of ketones when he administered a lethal dose of a chemotherapy drug into fasting mice and found it had little effect. Yet, initially healthy well-fed mice sickened and died. This protective effect is seen with exposure to other drugs as well. In neurological research, scientists use lab animals to test various treatments. In Parkinson's disease research, lab animals are treated with a synthetic heroin-like drug called MPP+ that destroys the dopamine-producing cells in the brain, causing the same symptoms as Parkinson's disease. A similar process is followed by scientists studying Alzheimer's disease. The amyloid protein, Abeta(1-42), is a substance that accumulates in the brains of Alzheimer's patients and destroys memory. A synthetic version is administered to lab animals to cause dementia. Ketones have been shown to block the harmful effects of both drugs, preserving normal brain cell function.[6] Another toxic drug rendered harmless by ketones is kainic acid, a potent neurotoxin used in medical research to cause seizures and brain cell damage. However, when fasting lab animals are exposed to kainic acid they suffer little or no harm.[7]

Aluminum phosphide (ALP) is a poison used for rodent control. It has also been used as a means to commit suicide. There is no known antidote and no effective treatment. ALP poisoning is almost always fatal. However, physicians in India have discovered a solution. When presented with a patient suffering from ALP poisoning, it has been found that feeding them coconut oil can block the toxic effects of the poison and bring about a complete recovery in most cases.[8] The reason coconut oil is so effective is that it is naturally ketogenic and is quickly converted into ketones in the body, raising blood ketone levels and neutralizing the poison.

There are many more natural and manmade toxins that are rendered harmless by ketones. If you would like to learn more about the amazing detoxifying effects of ketones, I recommend reading my book *Ketone Therapy: The Ketogenic Cleanse and Anti-Aging Diet.*

In addition to blocking the detrimental effects of toxins, ketones substantially lower free-radical or oxidative stress, preserving vital antioxidant nutrients such as vitamins A, C, D, and E that are important for healthy immune function. Ketones upregulate genes that produce powerful antioxidant enzymes such as glutathione, catalase, and superoxide dismutase, which help with the detoxification of free radicals and other toxic substances. Ketones set into motion processes that increase the production of white blood cells in the bone marrow, increasing the army of immune cells available to battle infection, toxins, and abnormal cells. Ketones activate neurotrophic factors, special proteins that regulate cell function, repair, and growth.

When toxins flood into the bloodstream from fasting or ketogenic dieting, ketones act as a safety net to prevent harm. The poisons are neutralized and quickly flushed out of the body. This is part of the cleansing process associated with fasting. It is also the primary cause of what is known as the *healing crisis*.

We are continually exposed to toxins in our life and environment. For this reason, no matter how clean our diet, we can benefit greatly from keto cycling. Continually going through the keto-fasting cycle will keep our bodies clean and healthy inspite of the toxins surrounding us. This is yet another reason to continue cycling in and out of ketosis.

THE HEALING CRISIS

In the 19th century doctors noticed that when patients went on a fast they often experienced a variety of unpleasant symptoms associated with the cleansing or detoxification process. They called this a healing crisis—"healing" because the body is cleansing and becoming healthier, "crisis" because it is a time of discomfort as toxins are purged from the body. The healing crisis is a natural cleansing reaction that is activated when the body is in ketosis. This is what many people call the "keto flu."

If you have lived most of your life on ultra-processed, packaged foods you will likely experience a healing crisis when you go on a fast or a ketogenic diet. The healing crisis is the most dramatic part of the cleansing process. You may feel great for a while and then come down sick—headaches, stomach cramps, skin eruptions, aches and pains throughout the body. This cleansing crisis may occur within a few days after you start a ketogenic diet or may not show up for several weeks or months. The crisis may repeat itself several times followed by periods of increasing feelings of well-being and improved health. Some people never experience a full-blown healing crisis. The healing crisis can manifest itself as a minor reaction that goes completely unnoticed or appear as if you had the flu or some other infection.

This is an area of confusion for many people. After eating healthy foods they would expect to get better, not sick. The diet is supposed to make them healthy! Why are they getting sick? These symptoms of illness are actually an indicator of improving health.

Many of the accumulated toxins we encounter in our day-to-day lives are trapped in fatty tissues. As dysfunctional protein and fatty tissue are dissolved and converted into energy during a fast or ketogenic diet, this debris is released into the bloodstream, where it is neutralized by ketones or the immune system and expelled from the body through any or all of the eliminating organs—skin, bowel, lungs, liver, and kidneys. Ketones are essential in neutralizing these toxins so that they are far less harmful. Their presence, however, may still cause reactions—symptoms.

This heavy release of toxins into the bloodstream and their removal from the body can bring on symptoms resembling a sickness. The symptoms will vary according to the materials being discarded, the condition of the organs involved in the elimination, your level of health, and the quality of your diet. You may experience some constipation, occasional diarrhea, coated tongue, frequent urination, nervousness, irritability, depression, fever, mucus discharge, cramps, headaches, muscle pain, skin rashes, swelling, nausea, canker sores, fever blisters, excess gas, tiredness, etc. You may experience discharges from every orifice, as the body purges impurities from the system. This is nature's way of cleansing the body.

One of the biggest misconceptions people face with the healing crisis is the belief that they have come down with the flu or caught some hideous infection (i.e., a disease crisis). If they go to a doctor who is not familiar with this aspect of natural healing, the doctor will likely diagnose it as an allergy or an infection and may prescribe antibiotics or other drugs which will suppress the healing process. Although the drugs may bring temporary relief from the symptoms, the cleansing process will be halted and toxins will remain in the body to be reabsorbed into the tissues.

There is an important difference between symptoms of the disease process and those of the healing process. The first is the result of the body succumbing to disease and the latter is the result of the body overcoming disease. The body has become strong enough to purge toxins and latent microbes from the tissues and, although symptoms of illness manifest themselves, the body is now strong enough to overcome the problem and eliminate the poisons. The organs of elimination have become stronger and energy levels have increased. Although this heavy release of toxins into the bloodstream might otherwise be harmful, ketones neutralize them, greatly weakening their toxic effects.

These symptoms are part of a curing process and are constructive. Don't try to stop them with medication. Natural herbal supplements, however, may be beneficial and can even speed healing, but they are not necessary. Let nature take its course. The symptoms generally will last only a day or two, but can hang on for a week or so. Unless absolutely necessary, no drugs should be taken during this time as the body is trying to eliminate toxins. Taking drugs will only hamper the elimination process and just add more toxins into your system. Do not eat any food or beverages sweetened with low-calorie or zero-calorie sweeteners of any type, as they will depress ketone production and cause symptoms to intensify. If symptoms arise, look on the positive side, it means you are ridding yourself of harmful toxins and excess fat and becoming healthier.

A single healing crisis may not purge all the toxins that have accumulated inside you over the years. You will not experience a healing crisis every time you fast or go on a ketogenic diet. You may never experience a significant cleansing reaction, or you may have them multiple times. It varies from person to person. The more often you cycle in and out of ketosis, the less likely you are to experience a major healing crisis, because after each cycle you become cleaner and healthier.

Symptoms can manifest themselves in any number of ways. If you have had problems with psoriasis, when you first start your diet, it may greatly improve the condition, although not completely clear it up. You may be relatively free of skin problems for a couple of months and feel the new way of eating is slowly working. Then, red, itching flaking skin will suddenly reappear and become as bad, if not worse, than it has ever been before, even though your diet has improved. Your first thought is that you are having a resurgence of the skin problems you've had for years. It may last a week or more, but then clear up completely, along with the dandruff problem you have had for the past 20 years. After this you will feel and look great. The dry flaky skin rash was the body's way of ridding itself of toxins.

If you have had dental problems, your teeth may hurt. You may encounter stabbing pain extending down to the nerve and feel as if it is infected. The body is healing; you don't need to have dental work at this time. Your teeth are removing bacteria, inflammations, etc., and although swelling may occur, and it may hurt to chew, it will heal on its own in a few days.

Longstanding joint pain may subside somewhat at first, then intensify for awhile, then go away completely; sinus problems or allergies may intensify and then fade in the same fashion. Many chronic conditions may improve for awhile, then briefly get worse before getting significantly better. And yet, some problems gradually just fade away without much notice.

You will continue to feel good for a time and then suddenly become tired and nauseous for a few days. When discomforting symptoms leave, you will feel better than you did before. Still later, you may have a headache, diarrhea, or a fever, but in a day or two you will feel better. Some healing crises are rather mild and may go unnoticed. Others may be quite severe and require bed rest for a few days. This is how recovery works. The first cleansing crisis is often the worst, with each succeeding reaction being milder and of shorter duration than the one before. The body becomes purer, stronger, and healthier with longer periods of symptom-free health, until you reach a level where you are relatively free of symptoms and illness.

No two people are alike. Everyone eats differently and has different genetic makeup and lifestyle. Everyone has different levels of health when they start on the program. The symptoms you encounter, their frequency, and their severity will be completely different from anyone else's. So you can't compare yourself with others.

During a crisis there is often an absence of appetite and an onset of tiredness. Drink plenty of clean water and get plenty of rest. Eat lightly, if at all. If you have no hunger, do not eat. Liquid, however, is vital to cleansing because water flushes out the toxins.

The first healing crisis will come according to the health of the individual. A young person may have a crisis after only a couple of weeks, while for an elderly person it may take a few months. Older people have a buildup of many more years of poor living habits to correct than younger ones. So, generally, the older you are, the more severe and more frequent crises will be.

Some people, when they experience their first healing crisis, think it's a disease crisis and give up because they believe the diet didn't work and just made them sicker. You can't expect to clean 40 years of junk and rebuild an entire body in just a few weeks. While detoxing, you do not grow older and sicker, but younger and healthier. You may see improvements in your health almost immediately. The longer you cycle in and out of ketosis the healthier you will be. If you return to habits that burden the body with poisons and pollution, good health cannot be maintained.

7

Low-Calorie Sweeteners

SUGARS AND SUGAR SUBSTITUTES
Sugar

It is generally believed, and rightly so, that sugar is addictive, promotes weight gain, rots our teeth, causes diabetes, increases the risk of cardiovascular disease, feeds cancer, accelerates aging of the brain, and is associated with various other health problems. One of the reasons why the ketogenic diet has proven so successful in reducing weight and improving overall health is that it totally eliminates sugar. Sugar in all of its many forms is off-limits. It doesn't matter if it is a so-called natural sweetener like honey or a highly processed product like table sugar (sucrose), the effects are basically all the same and cause much of the same health problems.

Sugar comes in many forms with various names that can be confusing. When you look at an ingredient label, sugar can be listed multiple times without you realizing it since many of the names are unfamiliar, such as maltodextrin and dextrin. The names of some types of sugar end with *–ose*, such as lactose, maltose, and glucose. If you see a word you are unfamiliar with ending in *–ose*, it most likely is some type of sugar. Following is a list of some of the many different names for sugar to look for on labels.

agave
barley malt
brown rice syrup
coconut sugar
corn syrup
date sugar
dextrin
dextrose
dulcitol
fructose
fruit juice
glucose
high fructose corn syrup
honey

lactose
levulose
maltodextrin
maltose
maple sugar
maple syrup
molasses
palm sugar
saccharose
sorghum
sucrose
treacle
turbinado
xylose

Sugar Substitutes

Since sugar is off-limits, there is a tendency to replace it with various sugar substitutes. There are many names which are used to describe these products: low-calorie sweeteners, zero-calorie sweeteners, nonnutritive sweeteners, and artificial sweeteners. Most of these terms are interchangeable. There are two major classes of low-calorie sugar substitutes: nutritive and nonnutritive. Nutritive sweeteners contain some calories. Sugar alcohols fit into this category. Nonnutritive sweeteners supply no calories. They are often referred to as zero-calorie or artificial sweeteners.

Sugar alcohols are not as sweet as sucrose but have fewer calories and, therefore, are often used as sugar substitutes. There are a number of different sugar alcohols. Most of them, but not all, end in *-itol*, such as sorbitol and mannitol. Following is a list of sugar alcohols:

erythritol
hydrogenated starch hydrolysates (HSH)
isomalt
lactitol
maltitol
mannitol
sorbitol
xylitol

Nonnutritive sweeteners are sugar substitutes that provide no calories, therefore have no nutrient value, but are many times sweeter than sugar (sucrose). Because of their lack of calories and high level of sweetness, they have been heavily promoted as harmless or at least safer alternatives to sugar. Following is a list of the most common nonnutritive sweeteners:

acesulfame K
advantame
aspartame
monk fruit extract
neotame
saccharin
stevia
sucralose

NONNUTRITIVE SWEETENERS
Sweeteners Promote Obesity, Diabetes, and Cardiovascular Disease

Beverages are the most commonly used products sweetened with nonnutritive sweeteners. Studying beverage consumption has provided insight into the consequences of using low-calorie sweeteners in place of sugar-sweetened products. You would think that reducing sugar intake by replacing sugar-sweetened beverages with products sweetened with nonnutritive sweeteners would lead to weight loss and better overall health, however, just the opposite has happened.

A study from researchers at Boston University School of Medicine, found that drinking at least one diet beverage daily puts a person at three times the risk of stroke and dementia compared to someone who drinks less than one a week.[1]

Researchers at the University of Texas examined the relationship between sugar-free beverage consumption and long-term weight gain in a group of about 5,000 subjects. They found that after 7 to 8 years, those consuming an average of three sugar-free sodas per day had double the risk of being overweight or obese than those who drank regular soda. You might think that those who already had weight issues were more likely to consume the sugar-free sodas; however, this was not the case here because all the subjects were normal weight at the beginning of the study.[2] The researchers summarized their results by stating, "These findings raise the question whether artificial sweetener use might be fueling—rather than fighting—our escalating obesity epidemic."

In another study involving children and adolescents 6 to 19 years of age, researchers found a correlation between being overweight and drinking sugar-free soda. The relationship between weight and soda consumption was much weaker in those who drank regular soda, sugary fruit drinks, and other beverages, demonstrating again that diet soda is worse than sugar-sweetened beverages.[3]

According to a study published in the *Canadian Medical Association Journal,* individuals who routinely consume nonnutritive sweeteners may have an increased risk for long-term weight gain, obesity, high blood pressure, and heart disease. Evidence also suggests nonnutritive sweeteners could have negative effects on metabolism, alter gut bacteria, and increase appetite (promoting increased calorie consumption).[4]

The study examined the data from 37 previous studies that tracked the cardiovascular and metabolic health of more than 400,000 people who used nonnutritive sweeteners. The people weren't losing weight. In fact, the longer studies—which observed the participants for up to 10 years—noted that they were instead gaining weight, and they were more likely to be obese and have high blood pressure, diabetes, heart disease, and other health issues compared to those who did not use nonnutritive sweeteners (e.g., those who drank sugar-sweetened beverages). In other words, nonnutritive sweeteners had a greater adverse effect on health than did sugar.

It appears that nonnutritive sweeteners, which are promoted as a means to help us lose weight and keep the weight off and to prevent diabetes, are actually doing just the opposite and may be fueling our obesity epidemic and contributing to the soaring rise of type 2 diabetes. In the 1990s, fewer than 10 percent of the population used nonnutritive sweeteners. By 2008, more than 30 percent of Americans reported daily use of nonnutritive sweeteners. Today, that number has increased to over 50 percent.[5] Currently there are literally thousands of diet beverages and foods on the market. The increased use of nonnutritive sweeteners has mirrored the dramatic rise in obesity and type 2 diabetes.

Why Sugar Substitutes Cause Weight Gain

The Canadian study mentioned above substantiates the results of a number of other recent studies.[6-8] According to an Australian study published in the journal *Cell Metabolism*, nonnutritive sweeteners can stimulate appetite, leading to increased calorie consumption of up to 30 percent, thus promoting weight gain and other metabolic problems.[9] Additionally, the University of Sydney researchers found that the chronic consumption of nonnutritive sweeteners promoted hyperactivity, insomnia, glucose intolerance (insulin resistance), a more intense perception of sweetness, an increase in appetite, and greater total calorie consumption.

"We found that inside the brain's reward centers, sweet sensation is integrated with energy content. When sweetness versus energy is out of balance for a period of time, the brain recalibrates and increases total calories consumed," says Associate Professor Greg Neely, a co-author of the study. To put it simply, the sweeteners essentially cause the brain to send a message that not enough energy has been consumed, triggering a kind of starvation response that makes food taste even better.

When ordinary sugar is eaten, dopamine is released in the brain and blood sugar levels rise, causing a secondary stimulation to produce more dopamine. When eating nonnutritive sweeteners, dopamine produces the initial sensation of pleasure, but the second effect doesn't occur because sugar-free sweeteners do not increase blood sugar levels. As a result, the body sends signals requesting more food and more calories to compensate.

Another study, published in the *American Journal of Public Health*, found that people who were overweight or obese ate more when they drank nonnutritive sweetened diet beverages. This kind of drink was linked to increased energy intake ranging from 88 calories per day for overweight participants to 194 calories for obese participants.[10]

Studies have shown that it doesn't matter what type of nonnutritive sweetener is used, whether it is aspartame or stevia, the effects are essentially the same: weight gain and increased risk of diabetes and other metabolic problems.[11] It is the sweetness combined with the lack of corresponding calories, not the particular chemical makeup of the sweetener, that causes the problem. Therefore, any nonnutritive or zero-calorie sweetener will increase appetite and promote weight gain and all of its accompanying problems.

Nonnutritive Sweeteners Increase Risk of Diabetes in Just Two Weeks

A recent study has shown that nonnutritive sweeteners not only increase the risk of type 2 diabetes but can do so after just a few weeks of use.[12] The researchers gave healthy volunteers nonnutritive sweeteners, sucralose or acesulfame K, equal to that of drinking 1.5 liters of diet soda every day. Tests at the end of the two week study period revealed that the sweeteners altered the subjects' glucose metabolism, causing elevated blood glucose and insulin levels. The study found that just two weeks use of nonnutritive sweeteners was enough to cause changes in the volunteers' ability to properly manage their blood sugar, setting them on the path to developing diabetes.

This discovery is in line with earlier research that had found that nonnutritive sweeteners promote obesity and insulin resistance in animals as well as humans. In one study using 7 volunteers, glucose intolerance was discovered in 4 of the subjects in less than 7 days.[13] It is becoming clearly evident that nonnutritive sweeteners are far worse than sugar.

Childhood Obesity Starts in the Womb

The adverse effects of nonnutritive sweeteners are even seen in the children of women who use these sweeteners during pregnancy. The incidence of childhood obesity has more than doubled in the last 30 years. One-third of children in the US are now overweight or obese. Part of this problem is due to children consuming foods and beverages sweetened with nonnutritive sweeteners. Another part of the problem is the consumption of nonnutritive sweeteners during pregnancy, which greatly increases the risk of a child becoming obese.

In a study published in the *Journal of the American Medical Association Pediatrics,* researchers examined 3,033 mothers and their children. More than a quarter of the women consumed nonnutritive sweetened beverages during pregnancy. There was no association between nonnutritive sweetener use and weight at birth; however, after one year infants whose mothers consumed nonnutritive sweeteners were more likely to be overweight.[14] This effect was not due to maternal body mass index, diet quality, total energy intake, or other obesity risk factors. There was no association with an increased risk of being overweight if the mother consumed sugar sweetened beverages. The reason for the increased infant weight was attributed to the mother's consumption of zero-calorie sweeteners during pregnancy.

Nonnutritive sweeteners are known to alter the gut microbiome, shifting the microbiota toward populations that tend to promote weight gain and metabolic disturbances. During delivery, whatever type of microbiota inhabits the mother's digestive tract and birth canal will be passed on to the infant. Therefore, the infant will acquire the type of bacteria that promotes weight gain, leading to weight problems later on.

As more evidence is accumulating, it is becoming increasingly evident that nonnutritive sweeteners are causing more harm than good and are not suitable substitutes for sugar.

SWEET ADDICTION

The biggest challenge most people face when they start a ketogenic diet is overcoming sugar addiction. Just about anyone who has been eating the typical Western diet is addicted to sugar to some degree. We all love our sweets, whether they are in the form of desserts and candy, are disguised as meals like pancakes and syrup, muffins and coffee, toaster pastries, breakfast cereals, or are in the form of snacks like trail mix and energy bars. Giving up all these foods, even if only for a few weeks, is a challenge.

Sugar addiction is not a consequence of the unique chemical makeup of sugar. Any sweet tasting substance can cause sugar addition, whether it is sugar or aspartame. A more accurate name for sugar addiction is "sweet" addiction. It is the sweet taste that we become addicted to, not the sugar itself. When we eat any sweet substance, be it sugar or erythritol, it activates sweet taste sensors in our mouths and throats (yes, we have sweet taste sensors in our throats), that send signals to our brain, stimulating pleasure centers. These are the same areas of the brain stimulated by cocaine and heroin, and this response is why sugar can be so addicting.

Knowing that sugar is highly addictive, marketing geniuses have identified a golden opportunity to manipulate this addiction to their advantage, targeting low-carb and ketogenic dieters. The plan? Offer them all of their favorite sweet foods and desserts sweetened with low-calorie sweeteners. These sugar substitutes contain little or no carbohydrate and provide almost no calories, making them appear to be keto friendly. These sweeteners give keto dieters permission to eat all of their favorite junk foods just as they used to. Consequently, their diet ends up loaded with low-quality foods that aren't really that much different from what they used to eat—the types of foods that made them fat and sick in the first place.

There are keto muffins, waffles, syrup, cakes, crackers, chips, candy bars, ice cream—the list goes on and on. All of these types of foods were once forbidden on a ketogenic diet, but now with the miracle of low-calorie sweeteners have been embraced by many. When sweetened foods like this are available, people tend to eat more of them and far fewer vegetables. Nutrient-rich vegetables seem to get pushed out of the diet.

Unfortunately, many authors and keto diet promoters have fallen into this trap and promote the use of sugar substitutes. Many even sell these products or sell cookbooks loaded with sweetened foods and desserts. Who couldn't resist a book titled *Keto Desserts* filled with delectable pictures of all your favorite indulgences? All foods sweetened with sugar substitutes are anti-ketogenic and fuel sweet addiction. Sweet addiction is the number one reason why people fail to stick with their diets, including the ketogenic diet. The allure of sweets pulls at them until they succumb. The ketogenic diet is an excellent way to break sweet additions. It can do it in a matter of days, but in order to be successful you need to abandon *all* sweets, including foods containing sugar substitutes.

When people follow a ketogenic diet, even if they use sweeteners, they will benefit because they have abandoned many poor quality foods and reduced their carbohydrate intake, which improves blood sugar levels and other health markers. The problem is that they will not see all of the benefits that they could have if they had cut out all sweeteners. Some may even become discouraged and quit because the excess weight didn't come off as anticipated. Their sweet addiction is still active, so the allure of favorite treats leads them into temptation and eventually abandoning the diet.

ANTI-KETOGENIC EFFECT

All low-calorie sweeteners are anti-ketogenic. Some are more potent than others, but they can all knock you out of ketosis or greatly reduce your blood ketone levels. If you are trying to get into ketosis, sweeteners will make it much harder, forcing you to restrict your total carbohydrate intake to as little as 20 grams or so just to get into a moderate state of ketosis. Some people who find it difficult to get into ketosis blame it on the assumption that they are just more "carbohydrate sensitive" than others—a consequence of poor genes or a lifetime of improper eating. Generally, this is not the case. The more likely reason is the consumption of sugar substitutes. I heard one person lament that he was very carbohydrate sensitive and had to limit his carb intake to about 20 grams daily to get into ketosis, but he had no reservations about drinking 3 or 4 cans of diet cola daily. Even though diet beverages may contain no calories or carbs, they are not compatible with the ketogenic diet.

This situation is bad because the carbohydrates that are generally removed from the diet to get down to 20 grams or less are the most nutritious ones—vegetables. The carbohydrates that are consumed are those that are commonly eaten with sugar substitutes—low-carb breads, sweets, soda, and desserts—essentially, keto junk foods.

Sugar substitutes are found in a variety of products, not just foods. They are used to sweeten sugar-free gum, toothpaste, mouthwash, breath mints, and even vitamin and herbal supplements. You need to read the labels on every product you put into your mouth. This is important because even just the taste of something sweet can be powerful enough to knock you out of ketosis.

You might question whether simply brushing your teeth with a xylitol-sweetened toothpaste would have any significant effect, especially since you aren't swallowing any, but it does. The tiny fraction of a drop of xylitol or sucralose contained in a single pea-sized dab of toothpaste can knock you completely out of ketosis.

Longtime ketogenic researcher Dr. John Freeman relates in his book *The Ketogenic Diet: A Treatment for Epilepsy*, the story of Michelle, a child he was treating for epilepsy with the ketogenic diet. She was doing very well on the diet throughout the winter and spring, with a marked decrease in seizure frequency. In the summer, the family often went to their summer home at the beach on weekends. They would arrive on Friday, and by Saturday Michelle's ketone levels would be low and her seizures would dramatically increase. Her parents carefully checked everything she ate and turned the house over, looking for anything in their environment that could have knocked her out of ketosis. They found nothing.

With the help of a nurse at Johns Hopkins Hospital, they went over everything they did on Friday and Saturday. "When we arrived at the beach, we lathered Michelle with suntan lotion," they told the nurse. Aha! They checked the sunscreen lotion label and it contained sorbitol—a sugar alcohol. Enough of the sorbitol was absorbed through Michelle's skin to affect her ketone levels and her seizure threshold. After switching to a sorbitol-free sunscreen lotion, Michelle had no further problems.

Dr. Robert Atkins wrote about similar experiences in his book *Dr. Atkins' New Diet Revolution*. He reported that when people used toothpaste sweetened with xylitol—another sugar alcohol—it would kick them out of ketosis.

I have witnessed the same reaction with the use of stevia, and for this reason I do not recommend it. I used to use stevia thinking it to be a better option to artificial sweeteners and sugar alcohols because it is promoted as a "natural" sweetener. However, after seeing its anti-ketogenic effects firsthand, I was compelled to investigate the matter in detail, reading every published study I could find on it. To my surprise, I discovered that stevia was no better than sucralose or any other zero-calorie or artificial sweetener. Not only was it anti-ketogenic, but it was also associated with numerous health issues.

One of the universal problems with low-calorie sweeteners is that they *all* disrupt the gut microbiome and shift it toward an unhealthy direction that promotes obesity, insulin resistance, and diabetes. The reason for this has nothing to do with their particular chemical makeup, it is all about their stimulating effects on taste sensors. The sweet taste combined with the absence of corresponding calories causes chaos in our digestive tract. The sweet taste triggers the release of hormones and prepares the digestive tract to receive a certain amount of calories. However, if the sweet taste is triggered by a low-calorie sweetener, the digestive tract never receives the calories it is anticipating. This messes with our normal digestive processes, leading to a series of undesirable side effects that can promote gut dysbiosis, weight gain, and insulin resistance.

THE DARK SIDE OF STEVIA EXTRACT

Since its approval as a food additive and sweetener by the FDA in 2008, stevia has become the most popular sugar substitute among health-conscious individuals. Currently, it is found in over 1,000 food products, many of which are promoted as keto friendly. However, stevia is one of the most insidious food ingredients you can use because it creates a false sense of compliance to the ketogenic diet. People love it because it gives them an excuse to maintain their sweet addiction and enjoy all their favorite junk foods with the mistaken belief that it is doing them no harm. Some people have become so enamored with it that when I tell them the truth about it, they react as if I had just insulted their mother. The sad truth is that stevia is just as harmful as any other nonnutritive sweetener and should never be included in a ketogenic diet. The same can be said about monk fruit extract as well. It, too, has no place in a ketogenic diet.

Stevia is marketed as a harmless, and even healthy, herbal sweetener derived from a plant rather than from some chemist's laboratory. It's natural, we are told, so it has to be good. As such, it has been embraced as the sweetener of choice for those choosing a low-carb or keto lifestyle.

Just because something comes from a plant does not make it wholesome or harmless. There are many natural substances that are poisonous or otherwise harmful. Have you ever experienced the consequences of touching the leaf of a poison ivy plant or felt the pain of stinging nettle? Many poisons, such as cyanide and ricin, are derived from plants. Many dangerous drugs also come from plants.

Simply because stevia is derived from a plant does not make it harmless, let alone healthful.

Stevia marketers would like you to believe that the product sold as a sweetener in stores and used as a food additive is simply an herb. Nothing can be further from the truth. The sweetener that is sold in stores shares no resemblance to the stevia plant. In fact, these sweeteners should not even be called stevia, but by their chemical names rebaudioside A and stevioside. It's all a part of the misconception that stevia marketers use to deceive the public. The stevia sweetener you buy in the store cannot be called an herb or even a natural product; it is a highly processed, refined, purified chemical. The sweetness of stevia comes from chemicals called steviol glycosides. In the refining process, all of the vitamins, minerals, antioxidants, essential oils, and other plant components are stripped away, leaving purified steviol glycosides. Some manufactures purify their products into individual steviol glycosides, primarily rebaudioside A and stevioside.

Stevia is no more natural than is sugar or cocaine. Sugar is extracted and refined from sugar beets. Cocaine is extracted and refined from coca leaves. Likewise, stevia sweetener is extracted and refined from stevia leaves. To call stevia an "herbal" sweetener is like calling sugar a "vegetable" sweetener because it comes from beets. Like sugar and cocaine, purified stevia extract forms a white crystalline powder. It has no resemblance to the original herb in any way, shape, or form. It is more like a drug than an herb. Its most potent drug-like effect is its sweetness, which is 200 to 300 times sweeter than sugar.

Stevia has been heavily promoted as harmless and even healthy with a sweetness like sugar but without any of the health risks. A natural sweetener that is harmless, as well as healthy, is a dream come true for those looking for better alternatives to sugar and sugar substitutes. In fact, it seems too good to be true. As the saying goes, "If it sounds too good to be true, it probably is." This is apparently the case with stevia as well.

Although stevia promoters like to claim that the sweetener has no known harmful effects; this is simply not true. Human clinical studies have documented various side effects that include nausea, abdominal discomfort, muscle pain, headache, fatigue, and dizziness.

Additionally, dermatitis, joint pain, digestive distress, mouth sores, vertigo, miscarriages, weight gain, glucose intolerance, and allergic reactions have been reported. Evidence also suggests that stevia may cause problems that lack any clear or immediate signs of symptoms such as infertility, DNA damage, gut microbiome dysbiosis, and damage to the heart, liver, and kidneys.[15] Adverse reactions to stevia may be far more common than most people realize. Since we have repeatedly been told that stevia is harmless, when people do experience an adverse reaction they tend to attribute it to something else. Some effects are minor and are generally ignored, while others can be serious and even potentially deadly, as was the case with two-year-old Mason, who was rushed to the hospital after consuming water sweetened with stevia.[16] In one double blind study, 13 percent of 60 subjects taking an extract of purified steviol glycosides experienced side effects troubling enough to report to the investigators; in three cases the effects were so severe the subjects were forced to withdraw from the study.[17] According to the study data, one out of every five people who use stevia may suffer some type of *noticeable* adverse reaction. Whether they recognize that it is caused by stevia is another matter.

Joseph Nelson, MD, has seen the detrimental effects of stevia in both his life and the lives of his patients. Dr. Nelson is a family physician specializing in integrative medicine. He spent 13 years with the FDA working on drug research, but when he refused to cover up adverse effects associated with a blood pressure medicine, he was fired as a whistleblower. His outspoken opposition to aspartame also landed him in hot water with the G. D. Searle company, the maker of NutraSweet, who tried unsuccessfully to sue him. When Searle threatened him, he told them he would love the opportunity for the publicity, so they backed down and withdrew the lawsuit. He worked in the supplement industry for awhile, then later went into private practice, merging conventional and natural medicine.

Dr. Nelson first became aware of the possible problem with stevia after he had a routine PSA test. This test measures the level of a protein called prostate-specific antigen (PSA) in the blood. High PSA levels indicate the possibility of serious problems such as prostate cancer, benign prostatic hyperplasia (enlarged prostate), or prostatitis. Men are encouraged to have the test done annually after the age of 50. Generally, a PSA reading of 4.0 ng/ml and lower is considered normal. If a man has a PSA above this, doctors often recommend a prostate biopsy to determine whether cancer is present. The higher the PSA level, the greater the risk of cancer. Surprisingly, Dr. Nelson's PSA numbers had suddenly risen from a stable and safe 2.0 to an incredible 19.6! Against his better wishes, he immediately made an appointment with an urologist to get a prostatic biopsy.

The next night, while he was lying in bed, he suddenly made the connection. He had added stevia into his diet during the year and he wondered, could that have been the problem? Over the next two weeks, he avoided all sources of stevia and then repeated the PSA test. It dropped to 8.2. Nothing else in his life during this time had changed. Stevia became his prime suspect.

At this point, he decided to run an experiment with his patients. He took every male patient with an elevated PSA and asked them to do a PSA test. He also looked for any evidence of stevia in their diet. Many people do not purposely add stevia to their foods but are still exposed to it as an ingredient in the foods, beverages, and supplements they consume. He removed all sources of stevia from these patients' diets for two weeks and again measured their PSA levels. He watched the abnormally elevated PSA levels drop at least 30 and usually 50 to 60 percent within the two weeks. One patient's PSA dropped from an incredibly high reading of 54 down to 12 within that short amount of time. He had never seen a response like this before. PSA levels are notoriously stubborn to move, but the removal of stevia from the patients' diets brought about an instant response. The connection was obvious.

One of his patients whose PSA level had been stable for years experienced a sudden rise. Dr. Nelson asked him if he used stevia or anything sweetened with it. He told him no. Dr. Nelson believed the patient was getting it somehow and told him to look for any source of stevia he might be exposed to at home. The patient began looking. It wasn't in any of his foods or beverages, not in any supplements, gum, or toothpaste, and he was about to give up when he read the label on a bottle of Losartan HCTZ—his blood pressure medication. There it was. Apparently, the drug maker coated the pills with stevia to make them taste better. Stevia can be in just about any product without you knowing it. It doesn't take much—even just the coating on a pill—to cause an effect, so any source can be significant.

Dr. Nelson's second experience with stevia occurred when one of his patients bought a 5 pound bag of the sweetener. The next day she suddenly developed a severe case of vertigo. She recognized the cause of her problem without the doctor's help. Soon afterward, Dr. Nelson had another patient come to him complaining of vertigo that had persisted for eight days. He told her to look for any food, supplement, or medication she was using that might contain stevia. She discovered that a brand of tea she used contained it. The manufacturer had just recently added it to their products without informing its customers. She stopped using the tea and her vertigo went away.

Dr. Nelson is a member of a group of local healthcare practitioners, mostly chiropractors and nutritionists,who regularly discuss current health issues. After telling them about his experience, they all told him that they were experiencing an epidemic of vertigo in their practices and that it was apparently due to stevia.

In his practice and being aware of the potential problems with stevia, Dr. Nelson has identified stevia as being involved with a variety of health issues including elevated PSA, bladder spasms, irritable bowel syndrome, vertigo, hypoglycemia, and most recently, chest pain and heart disease.

A woman came to his office complaining of anxiety, heart palpitations, and chest pain. He ran her through a series of tests, including an echocardiogram to evaluate the condition of her heart. The tests were all normal. He could not find anything wrong with her. He checked her diet and any supplements or medications she was using. She was taking a powdered magnesium dietary supplement with fruit flavoring and stevia. As soon as she stopped taking the supplement, her chest pain and associated symptoms immediately disappeared. It was also noted in retrospect that she was not having these problems during her vacations and travel because the powder was unwieldy to travel with and she was using tablets that did not contain stevia. After removing the stevia from her diet she no longer experienced the problem.

Dr. Nelson discovered that stevia may damage the heart. When your doctor orders blood tests, one of the markers that may be measured is a hormone called brain natriuretic peptide or BNP. Although the name of this hormone suggests that is associated with the brain, it is not. The name came about because it was originally identified in extracts of pig brain. BNP is secreted by the heart in response to stress and is used as a marker to evaluate risk of heart failure and, to a lesser extent, kidney disease. It is an especially reliable predictor of cardiovascular mortality in diabetics.

Heart failure doesn't necessarily mean the heart has stopped working entirely. Rather, it means it is not working properly so it doesn't fully support the body's need for blood and oxygen. Heart failure is serious and is one of the most common reasons for hospitalization of people over the age of 65. Over time, it can get worse and lead to death. Anything that can damage the heat can lead to heart failure, including coronary artery disease, heart attack, cardiomyopathy, high blood pressure, and diabetes.

When you have heart failure, your heart produces two related hormones: one called B-type natriuretic peptide (BNP) and the other N-terminal-pro-BNP (NT-proBNP). Levels of both hormones increase when heart failure gets worse and decrease when it gets better. A BNP blood test measures these two hormones. NT-proBNP in the range of 125-450 pg/mL is considered normal or mild to moderate stress; a reading above 450 pg/mL is an indication of heart failure or severe stress—not a good sign. Risk of cardiac arrest and death increases with increasing BNP levels.

Dr. Nelson discovered that stevia can have a direct effect on the heart as indicated by BNP levels. This was first revealed to him by a patient whose blood test showed a NT-proBNP level of 628 pg/mL—an indication of heart failure. Over the next 6 months, the patient pursued the standard drug treatment for heart failure. On the follow-up visit the patient's NT-proBNPlevel had risen to 699pg/mL, showing that her condition was getting worse. This suggested that she was doing something that was continuing to harm her heart despite the medications and treatment. On investigation, it was discovered that she was using a sweetened energy drink daily that contained stevia. She was instructed to stop using the product. Two months later she had another blood test. This time, her NT-proBNP level had dropped to 375 mg/mL—down into the normal range. This change occurred by simply discontinuing stevia, nothing else in her diet or lifestyle had changed.

This is significant because it suggests that stevia may be harmful to the heart. If you have had heart issues or are concerned about the health of your heart, it may be wise to avoid stevia and products containing it.

When I tell people about all of the potential health problems associated with stevia some skeptics respond with, "I've been using it for years and I haven't experienced any problems." However, how can they be sure, especially with something like heart disease? Keep in mind, the first symptom of heart disease that most people experience is a heart attack. There may be no noticeable symptoms until the damage is severe.

Dr. Nelson notes that we are repeating history. The same thing is beginning to happen that occurred after the introduction of aspartame. Promoters marketed aspartame as a harmless sweetener. Studies by the sweetener maker proved it. Yet, countless people experienced troubling adverse reactions. The battle raged on for years. Even today most doctors continue to claim that aspartame is safe and deny it has any harmful effect; people who say the opposite are often considered delusional. Informed people, however, know better. We are entering into a new war, this time with stevia. The food manufacturers and promoters selling the product are squaring off against any dissenting voice that dares to claim otherwise. Don't be fooled by food and supplement manufacturers or their clever marketing gimmicks. Their goal is to sell products, not to worry about your health.

8

Keto Myths, Mistakes, and Misconceptions

There are many myths, mistakes, and misconceptions regarding the ketogenic diet that are perpetuated on the internet, by the media, and even in books. Some of the mistakes people make are minor, others are more serious, and some are so severe that they significantly affect the results of the diet. Let's look at 24 of the most common myths and mistakes.

Myth 1: You Don't Need to Count Your Carb Intake

We tend to be lazy and try to take shortcuts. One of these shortcuts is to not keep track of daily net carbohydrate consumed, believing that simply eliminating grains, potatoes, fruit, and sweets is enough to get into ketosis. This is not the case. Many vegetables and even processed meats and dairy contain a substantial amount of carbohydrate that needs to be accounted for. You might be surprised how many carbs a particular product may contain. If you don't count your carbs, you have no idea how much you're eating.

We have no idea how much carbohydrate is in most foods, nor do we realize how quickly the amount can add up. This is particularly true for those people who are just beginning a low-carb or ketogenic diet. Estimating does not work. You must make the effort to count every gram of carbohydrate in every meal and snack you consume.

Most people can get into mild ketosis by limiting total carbohydrate intake to less than 50 grams a day, as long as protein consumption is also limited to 60 to 90 grams/day. To reach a moderate state of nutritional ketosis, daily net carbohydrate intake should be limited to about 30 grams. When you first start the diet you need to calculate your net carbs (total carbs minus fiber). In time, you will become familiar with the types of low-carb foods you like and how many carbs are in each meal. After you reach this point, you can get by with estimating your carb intake.

In order to glean all of the benefits of being in ketosis and switching in and out of ketosis, you absolutely need to get into ketosis in the first place. The only way to guarantee that you are in ketosis is to count your net carb intake and to measure your ketone levels using a urine, blood, or breath test.

Myth 2: Eating a High-Fat Diet Is Unhealthy

As much as 90 percent of the calories in the ketogenic diet come from fat. The ketogenic diet is not just a high-fat diet, but an *extremely* high-fat diet. For years The American Heart Association and other organizations have recommended that we limit our fat intake to no more than 30 percent of our calories. They make this recommendation based primarily on the now outdated lipid hypothesis of heart disease, assuming that eating much more than 30 percent fat would cause heart disease or other health problems.

Many people worry that blood cholesterol levels will skyrocket on the ketogenic diet. This is really not an issue to worry about. Cholesterol is not your enemy. Studies on cholesterol levels in patients following the ketogenic diet do show that, on average, total blood cholesterol levels often increase, but risk factors for heart disease (high blood pressure, HDL cholesterol, blood triglycerides, inflammation), actually improve, reducing the risk.

The high-fat ketogenic diet has been in use for nearly a century. For most of that time, those on the diet ate primarily saturated fats, the kind that dietitians today often tell us to avoid. Yet, after nearly a century of use with literally thousands of patients consuming a 60 to 90 percent fat diet for extended periods of time (years, in fact), the diet has caused no heart attacks or strokes. Indeed, just the opposite has happened. People have been healed from epilepsy, lost excess body fat, and experienced many additional health benefits.

Saturated fats generally raise HDL cholesterol, the so-called good cholesterol that helps protect against heart disease. Because your HDL increases, it may also raise your total cholesterol somewhat. This is okay. Total cholesterol is a very poor indicator of heart disease risk. The reason for this is that total cholesterol is the combined total of your HDL and LDL and VLDL, and you don't know how much of each makes up the total. This is why half of all those who suffer a heart attack have normal to below normal or even optimal total cholesterol levels. The increase in HDL could raise your total cholesterol, but this isn't the full picture. An increase in HDL affects your cholesterol ratio (total cholesterol/HDL) as well as total cholesterol, so you may still have a reduced risk of heart disease.

The ketogenic diet may also slightly raise your LDL cholesterol as well. LDL cholesterol has been labeled the "bad" cholesterol, the cholesterol that causes problems. However, we now know there are two types of LDL cholesterol: one that is large and buoyant and another that is small and dense. The large LDL cholesterol is another type of "good" cholesterol. The small LDL cholesterol is the one that is associated with increased risk of heart disease. On a ketogenic diet the large, beneficial LDL increases while the small, not so good LDL decreases. While total cholesterol may still increase, the change in cholesterol is protective against heart disease and beneficial.

The safety of high fat diets actually extends back thousands of years. A number of populations traditionally have survived and even thrived on diets supplying 60 to 90 percent of calories as fat. The most notable, perhaps, are the Inuit. The Inuit historically lived near the Arctic Circle from Alaska to Greenland, where edible vegetation was scarce. The traditional Inuit diet contained virtually no carbohydrate after weaning (milk contains some carbohydrate), relying totally on meat and fat for the rest of their lives. Yet, the Inuit were described by early arctic explorers as robust and healthy, free from the diseases of civilization such as heart disease, diabetes, dementia, and cancer, and living to an age equal to that of contemporary Americans and Europeans. The same can be said of the American Plains Indians before colonization by white settlers, the native Siberians (Buryat Mongols, Yakuts, Tatars, Samoyeds, Tunguses, Chukuhis, and others) of northern Russia, and the Maasai of Africa, all of whom thrived on extraordinarily high-fat diets. Their diets were not just high in fat but high specifically in saturated fat and cholesterol, yet heart disease was unheard of among them. Even today, those people who continue their traditional high-fat diets are remarkably free from the degenerative diseases that are so common in Western society. High-fat diets have withstood the test of time and have proven to be not only safe, but therapeutic.

Myth 3: You Can Lose Weight on the Ketogenic Diet without Restricting Calories

One of the major mistakes about keto for weight loss is that you can eat all you want and still lose weight. Many studies have shown that in comparison to a low-fat, calorie-restricted diet, a ketogenic diet without calorie restriction produces greater weight loss. When in ketosis, hunger is depressed, so a person can feel satisfied eating fewer calories than normal, and consequently, total calorie intake often declines somewhat. In contrast, a low-fat, high-carb diet is less satisfying and generally stimulates increased hunger.

For these reasons, people often get the idea they can eat as much as they want on a ketogenic diet, even three full meals a day, and the weight will easily melt off. You may lose a few pounds initially, but that is about all. If you are serious about weight loss, you must also consciously reduce your total calorie intake as well. Intermittent fasting can be of great benefit in your weight loss efforts.

Being in ketosis is a great aid in weight loss as it blunts hunger so that you can eat fewer calories without suffering from hunger pangs like you would with a low-fat diet. However, many people who believe they are following a ketogenic diet never really get into ketosis or remain in ketosis for long due to poor advice and misconceptions often perpetuated on the internet. If you are not actually in ketosis you will feel no significant decline in hunger. It takes 3 to 7 days on the ketogenic diet before you will get into a moderate state of ketosis. As you get into a deeper state of ketosis your hunger will decline.

Although hunger decreases dramatically, some people complain of hunger. Hunger is often caused by a lack of fat in the diet. Often people increase fat intake somewhat when they go keto, but they don't really know how much fat they are actually eating. This lack of understanding leads to them not eating nearly enough fat. You need to increase total fat intake to account for at least 60 percent of your daily calories. Adding more fat will help keep you from being hungry.

Also, hunger pangs may come not because you are actually hungry, but because you are thirsty. This is your body trying to tell you to drink something. Drinking a glass of water will provide you with needed water and ease your hunger pangs.

Another reason why you may feel hungry is if you use some type of sugar substitute in your foods or beverages. Sugar substitutes promote hunger and fuel sugar addiction. Eliminate them all. They do you no good and can cause a lot of harm.

Myth 4: The Ketogenic Diet Will Cause You to Lose Weight Even If You Are Underweight

Some normal weight or underweight people hesitate to try the ketogenic diet in fear that it might make them lose weight. When you first start the ketogenic diet, you may lose a little, but if you eat at the same frequency as you normally do and do not reduce the total amount of food you eat, you are not likely to lose any significant amount of weight. The diet should help you maintain a healthy weight.

Generally, people who are normal weight do not overeat or overindulge in sweets and baked goods (breads, cookies, pastries, etc.)—the primary contributors to overweight. Since these types of foods are not consumed in the ketogenic diet, eating preferences will not be that much different.

Underweight individuals can go on a ketogenic diet, but it is best that they not fast. They can still cycle in and out of ketosis by going keto for awhile and then feasting for awhile, alternating back and forth.

Myth 5: You Need to Stay On a Ketogenic Diet for Life to Benefit

Most people view diets as temporary means to achieve a goal, generally weight loss or to reduce risk factors for heart disease or some other chronic ailment. Once the goal has been reached, or the person tires of dieting, they go back to eating their favorite foods. In time, old eating habits return, along with the weight and health problems. The only way to maintain all of the benefits achieved from dieting is to maintain the diet indefinitely.

For this reason, many people assume that the ketogenic diet must also be maintained for life. Being in a continual state of nutritional ketosis is not recommended and is counterproductive. While the ketogenic diet can be tremendously helpful and improve insulin sensitivity, the benefits gradually decline over time. Being in ketosis for a prolonged period of time can make your more sensitive to carbohydrates and increase your risk of insulin resistance.

If you want to permanently improve your health and reduce the risk of chronic disease, you need to integrate the ketogenic diet as part of a lifestyle change. This would involve a permanent change in eating patterns, not strictly a ketogenic diet, but rather alternating from a normal mixed diet to a ketogenic diet, with intermittent fasting—keto cycling. The transition from glucosis to ketosis activates and deactivates genes, initiates cleansing and autophagy, and stimulates the development of new stem cells. All of which, removes old worn out cells and tissues and replaces them with new, functional cells and tissues, reduces the risk of chronic disease, and prolongs healthy lifespan. Cycling also makes the ketogenic diet something that can be incorporated into a permanent lifestyle change without the need to totally eliminate healthy, but higher-carb foods or the enjoyment of an occasional treat.

Myth 6: The Ketogenic Diet Is High in Protein

The misperception that the ketogenic diet is a high-protein diet is proclaimed all over the internet and in the media, so it is no surprise that many people are confused. Critics who do not take the time to actually learn anything about the diet believe it is simply a hyper-low-carb diet that is loaded with protein and fat. The diet is low-carb, but it is not high in protein. It is accurately defined as a diet that is very low in carbohydrate, very high in fat, with low to moderate protein—just enough protein to meet daily needs and no more. The reason why protein is limited is because as much as 58 percent of the protein you eat can potentially be converted into glucose, which can raise blood glucose levels. Elevated glucose levels block the formation of ketones. Eating too much protein can therefore prevent you from getting into or knock you out of ketosis. For these reasons, your protein intake should be modest. Fat calories, not protein, take the place of the carbohydrate that is removed.

Protein consumption should be limited to about 60 to 90 grams per day depending on your size and activity level. If you are small or inactive, 60 grams would be ample protein for you. If you are tall or physically active 90 grams is adequate. If you very physically active or involved in competitive sports, you may need to increase your protein intake to 120 grams or so.

Myth 7: Vegetable Oils Are the Healthiest Fats

One of the distinctive characteristics of the ketogenic diet is the high fat intake. Fat is what gives the body most of its energy and supplies bulk to foods to satisfy hunger. Since fat contributes some 60 to 90 percent of the calories consumed, it is important to choose the best type of fat.

Saturated fats have been demonized as the cause of heart disease and other health problems for so many years that it is difficult for some people to fully embrace them. On the contrary, vegetable oils have been promoted as heart friendly because they tend to lower total cholesterol. Vegetable oils come from plants, primarily seeds and legumes, and therefore, are considered healthier alternatives to animal fats. Consequently, there is a tendency to want to use polyunsaturated or monounsaturated vegetables oils in preference to saturated fats. This is a big mistake.

Polyunsaturated fatty acids are chemically unstable and highly vulnerable to oxidation. Exposure to heat, light, and oxygen cause them to oxidize and become rancid, producing destructive free radicals. Polyunsaturated fatty acids start to oxidize from the moment processing begins as they are exposed to heat, oxygen, and light. Oxidation continues as the oils are bottled, warehoused, shipped, and stored on grocery shelves. At home or in restaurants, the heat used in food preparation greatly accelerates oxidation. By the time the oils are consumed, they are loaded with harmful free radicals that can wreak havoc on our cells and tissues.

The most common vegetable oils—soy, canola, cottonseed, corn, and safflower oils—are produced from genetically engineered plants and heavily sprayed with pesticides and contain a high level of pesticide residue. Unless they are certified organic, they are genetically altered and heavily sprayed. For these reasons, all processed polyunsaturated vegetable oils should be avoided.

Monounsaturated fatty acids are chemically more stable than polyunsaturated fatty acids and are not as easily oxidized. They can withstand low to moderate cooking temperatures without excessive damage, but will still degrade with exposure to heat, light and oxygen. Olive oil is composed predominantly of monounsaturated fatty acids. Macadamia nut, almond, and avocado oils are also rich sources of monounsaturated fatty acids.

Saturated fatty acids are the most stable and resistant to oxidation. This is why they are the preferred fats for cooking and frying. Animal fats (butter, lard, beef tallow, duck fat, etc.) and tropical oils (coconut, palm, and palm kernel), are the richest source of saturated fatty acids.

124

No natural oil is composed purely of polyunsaturated, monounsaturated, or saturated fatty acids. They all contain a combination or mixture of the different fatty acids. All dietary oils contain saturated fatty acids as well as polyunsaturated fatty acids. We refer to an oil as being "polyunsaturated" if it is predominantly polyunsaturated. Soybean oil is composed of 61 percent polyunsaturated fatty acids, 24 percent monounsaturated fatty acids, and 15 percent saturated fatty acids, so it is considered a polyunsaturated oil. Palm oil is composed of 50 percent saturated fatty acids, 40 percent monounsaturated fatty acids, and 10 percent polyunsaturated fatty acids, so it is considered a saturated oil.

Because of the high amount of fat consumed on the ketogenic diet, you need to use the healthiest fats possible. This would be those that are predominately saturated—animal fats and tropical oils. They are the most stable and least likely to oxidize. Monounsaturated fats can also be used in moderation. They are more stable than polyunsaturated fats but less stable than saturated fats. Diets containing more than 10 percent total calories from polyunsaturated fatty acids greatly increase the risk of cancer, low immune function, blood disorders, hormonal imbalances, and other problems, so it is wise to keep your intake of polyunsaturated fatty acids to a minimum.

The most compatible natural fat to use with a ketogenic diet is coconut oil. Coconut oil is naturally ketogenic. When consumed, it automatically is converted into ketones. Other oils do not do this unless the body is already in a state of ketosis. Coconut oil can boost blood ketone levels, enhancing the effects of the diet. Coconut oil is also heat stable, making it an excellent cooking and frying oil. It also contains the least amount of polyunsaturated fatty acids of any dietary oil—only 2 percent.

Myth 8: A Low-Carb, High-Fat Diet Is the Same as a Ketogenic Diet

Although the ketogenic diet is low-carb, not all low-carb diets are ketogenic. Simply combining a lot of fat with a low-carb diet does not make it ketogenic. Most low-carb diets contain far too much protein to be ketogenic. The excess protein prevents the body from going into nutritional ketosis. If the diet does not induce nutritional ketosis, it is not ketogenic.

Also, many so-called low-carb diets do not restrict total carbohydrate intake enough to initiate ketosis. Carbohydrate intake for a typical unrestricted diet ranges between 50 to 60 percent of total calories. A diet that contains only 20 or 30 percent of calories from carbohydrate would, therefore, be considered low carb. However, for the diet to be ketogenic, carbohydrate would need to be restricted to less than about 10 percent of calories. In a 2,000 calorie diet, that would limit total carbohydrate intake to 50 grams or less.

The only way to tell if you are eating a diet that promotes nutritional ketosis is to measure you ketone levels. This can be done with urine test strips, blood test strips, or breath analyzer.

Myth 9: You Need High Blood Ketone Levels to Benefit

Some people have assumed that the higher the blood ketone levels are, the better. Research is being conducted to develop drugs that can increase ketone levels many times higher than what is possible from eating coconut or MCT oils. While some level of ketosis is necessary in order to see therapeutic effects, high blood ketone levels have not been shown to be any more effective than much lower levels. The idea that "more is better" isn't necessarily true when it comes to ketones. This is apparently the case with seizure control in epileptics. Measures of seizure protection and seizure incidence with ketones levels do not correlate.[1]

We always have measurable concentrations of ketones in our blood regardless of our diet. The concentration of beta-hydroxybutyrate (BHB), the primary ketone, is typically around 0.1 mmol/l (millimoles per liter). During starvation or prolonged fasting, BHB levels increase to 2 to 7 mmol/l, which is also the same level achieved on the classic ketogenic diet. Therapeutic levels of ketosis that are effective in treating Alzheimer's disease can be achieved with blood levels of BHB less than 0.5 mmol/l.[2] This level can easily be achieved by consuming a 2 tablespoon dose of coconut oil. Blood levels of ketones at about this level have shown to be just as effective as those which are many times higher and typically associated with the ketogenic diet.[3] High ketone levels are not necessary.

You can think of it like filling the gas tank of your car. The tank can be filled to the top with fuel, but the engine can only burn a little at a time. The amount of gas in the tank has no effect on the rate at which the engine can burn the fuel. As long as enough gas is available to keep the engine continually running, it doesn't matter how full the tank is. The same is true with ketones. Pumping the body with more ketones than it needs will have no additional benefit. Excess ketones are not stored, like fuel is in the gas tank, or like glucose (which is

126

stored as glycogen). Ketones have a short lifespan in the blood. If they are not used within a couple of hours, they are flushed out of the body in the urine. So a large influx of ketones into the bloodstream will end up being removed from the body and do absolutely no good.

Myth 10: Ketosis Is Potentially Dangerous

There is widespread confusion among both physicians and laypeople about the ketogenic diet and ketosis. Many doctors have voiced concerns about the use of nutritional ketosis, believing it can lead to acidosis—excessively low blood pH (too acidic). This belief is based on observations of a life-threatening condition sometimes seen in untreated type 1 diabetics called ketoacidosis. Ketones are slightly acidic. The presence of too many ketones can make the blood acidic, causing ketoacidosis, which can throw a person into a diabetic coma. Doctors learn about ketoacidosis in school but usually don't learn anything about nutritional ketosis or the ketogenic diet. For this reason, they tend to view any level of ketosis as a warning sign of ketoacidosis and often caution patients about ketogenic dieting.

Regardless of what you may hear from your doctor or read on the internet, following a ketogenic diet will not cause ketoacidosis. Nutritional ketosis is not the same as, nor even similar to, diabetic ketoacidosis. The former is a normal metabolic condition of the body that can be manipulated by diet. The latter is a disease state that generally only occurs in type 1 diabetics.

Insulin is required in order to transport glucose from the blood into the cells. Type 1 diabetics are unable to produce an adequate amount of insulin. For this reason, they require regular insulin injections. Ketoacidosis can occur after eating a high-carbohydrate meal. Without an injection of insulin, glucose cannot enter the cells and blood glucose levels can rise dangerously high. Not only is the high glucose level toxic, but without glucose, the cells literally begin to starve to death. This is a life-threatening situation that affects the brain, heart, lungs and all other organs. To prevent imminent death, the body shifts into crisis mode and begins frantically pumping ketones into the bloodstream to provide the cells the fuel they need to survive. Cells can absorb ketones without the aid of insulin. Since none of the cells are able to access the glucose, ketones are continually being pumped into the bloodstream as an alternative fuel source. Ketone levels rise so high, they cause the blood to become acidic, creating a state of acidosis.

Ketoacidosis occurs only in untreated type 1 diabetics and on very rare occasions in severe cases of alcoholism. It cannot be triggered by diet alone. Low-carb ketogenic diets produce ketone levels in the blood of about 1 to 2 mmol/l. Extended periods of complete fasting raise ketone levels to 5 to 7 mmol/l. This is as high as ketone levels from dietary manipulation get because the body carefully regulates ketone production. In ketoacidosis, however, ketone levels rise above 10 mmol/l. The body is fully capable of buffering the effects of ketones at fasting levels, but when they rise to 20 mmol/l or more, it is beyond the body's ability to handle.

Myth 11: Keto Test Strips Are Inaccurate and Unreliable

Urine test strips are the most economical and easiest method to measure your level of nutritional ketosis. You can get 50 test strips for just a few dollars. Some people have discouraged the use of urine test strips, claiming that they are inaccurate and to get a true measure of the level of ketones in your blood you need to use a blood monitor. These monitors can cost several hundred dollars, with each test strip costing another five dollars or more. The blood test measures the amount of the ketone beta-hydroxybutyrate or BHB and gives a digital value which is very accurate at the time of the test.

In contrast, the urine test strips measure another ketone, acetoacetate or AcAc. Both BHB and AcAc increase as blood sugar declines and provide a relative measure of total blood ketone levels. Although it looks impressive to get a digital reading using the blood test, you don't need this level of accuracy to see if you are in ketosis or not. The reason for monitoring your ketosis levels is simply to see if your diet has gotten you into ketosis and to approximately what level—trace, low, medium, high. That is all the data you need. This is what the urine test strips do for a very affordable price.

A study published in the journal *Diabetes Metabolism* in 2007 compared urine and blood ketone testing. The researchers performed both tests on 529 adult patients. They concluded that there was a reasonably good correlation between urine and blood ketone tests at lower levels that would typically measure nutritional ketosis, but poor correlation for high values that are needed to confirm ketoacidosis—a metabolic disorder where blood sugar levels are poorly controlled.[4] Since you are only measuring for nutritional ketosis and not for ketoacidosis, the urine test strips are adequate.

When you are in ketosis, your liver will continually be producing ketones and releasing them into your bloodstream. Once formed, ketones don't remain in the blood for long. If not consumed, they are filtered out by the kidneys and excreted in the urine. Therefore, if you are in ketosis, you will always be excreting excess ketones. If a urine test shows no measurable level of ketones, then you are not in ketosis.

Some people have found that after being in ketosis for awhile they suddenly are no longer in ketosis even though their diet has not significantly changed. In order to account for this anomaly the explanation given is that as soon as a person has become keto adapted (about 2 to 3 weeks), the body burns ketones so efficiently that ketones stop spilling into the urine and the test strips stop measuring ketones. However, no matter how well adapted to burning fat you become, your body does not stop excreting ketones. I have never seen anyone who was following the diet properly not have measurable ketones in their urine. The test strips have worked fine for people who have been in ketosis for many months and still give useful readings.

If a person is finding that the urine test shows no ketones, it means just that: ketone levels are too low to measure. That means something is wrong with the diet; the dieter is eating too many carbs, too much protein, using sugar substitutes, or doing something else that affects the ketone levels, such as using toothpaste or taking dietary supplements containing xylitol or other sweeteners.

You should be continually monitoring your level of ketosis. If not, you will not be able to tell if you slide out of ketosis even though you think your diet has not changed much. Slight changes over time may seem unnoticeable but can significantly alter your metabolism. Testing every day or two will keep you on track and alert you to unnoticeable changes in your diet, problem foods, supplements, medications, or body care products.

Myth 12: Low-Calorie Sweeteners Are Compatible with the Ketogenic Diet

Sugar substitutes, especially zero-calorie sweeteners, contain no carbohydrate and contribute no calories, and therefore, appear to be ideally suited to the ketogenic diet. If carbohydrate and calories were the only things you needed to worry about, that might be true. However, there are other problems with low-calorie sweeteners. All low-calorie sweeteners affect hormones and the gut microbiome in ways that promote weight gain and insulin resistance. More importantly, they are all anti-ketogenic. If you are in ketosis, they can kick you out. If you are trying to get into ketosis, they can prevent it. Even the smallest amount—a single drop is enough to have a significant effect. If you include low-calorie sweeteners in a ketogenic diet it will greatly reduce your liver's ability to produce ketones. If you use these sweeteners, in order to reach low to moderate levels of ketosis, you need to restrict carbohydrate intake substantially, to as little a 20 grams a day.

If you are in ketosis and begin to add sweetened foods, you can be kicked out of ketosis without even realizing it. This is one reason why you should be in the habit of always monitoring your level of ketosis with urine test strips or other testing methods.

Most of the types of foods that are consumed with sweeteners are junk foods with little nutritional value. Consuming these types of food displaces other, more nutritious foods from your diet. Thus using low-calorie sweeteners also decreases the nutritional content of the diet.

Low-calorie sweeteners can be hidden in a variety of products besides foods, including supplements, tea, medications, spices, gum, toothpaste, mouthwash, and lip gloss. You don't need to swallow it, just the taste of the sweetness can arrest ketone production.

Myth 13: Keto Convenience Foods Are Compatible with the Ketogenic Diet

Because of the popularity of low-carb and keto diets, many food manufacturers have developed low-carb foods that resemble popular higher-carb snacks, treats, and baked goods, which are essentially nothing more than keto junk foods.

Most of these foods are sweetened with sugar substitutes, which make them appear to be keto friendly. However, we know that all sugar substitutes are anti-ketogenic and promote hunger, overeating, and insulin resistance. Like any other junk food, keto junk foods are ultra-processed and low in nutrition. Although the ingredients may appear to be natural, many of the ingredients are highly processed and often use nuts, seeds, and oils that have gone rancid.

Eating keto junk foods that resemble the junk foods you used to eat isn't really changing your diet or eating habits. It is just substituting one unhealthy junk food with another. Eating these types of foods will push other, more healthy foods out of the diet. A proper ketogenic diet should focus on fresh vegetables, fruits, meats, eggs, dairy, and healthy fats and forgo processed convenience foods.

When you break your addiction to sweets and junk foods and begin eating a truly ketogenic diet, you will notice that fresh whole foods taste better. Vegetables, meats, and eggs seem to taste much better when you are on a ketogenic diet. You may even crave your vegetables! When you go keto, your sense of taste improves, foods become more flavorful, and you can taste the subtle sweetness in foods that you had never noticed before. At the same time, sugar cravings go away (as long as you are not eating sugar substitutes). Sweets no longer have control over you. You have control over them and can refuse them without a second thought.

Myth 14: Diet Soda and Coffee Are Keto Friendly

You need to keep in mind that the ketogenic diet was designed to mimic fasting. To accomplish this, carbohydrate and protein intake must be kept to a minimum. Fat is permissible because a fasting body uses fat as it primary source of fuel. Whether this fat comes from body stores or the diet doesn't matter, as the metabolic effects are the same. Therefore, any beverages you consume must not affect your metabolism either.

Water is by far the preferred beverage. Mineral water and unsweetened herbal tea may also be used. Other beverages are not compatible. This includes milk, juice, alcohol, black tea, coffee, and diet beverages. Milk has too high a carbohydrate content. A single cup (8 oz/236 ml) of whole milk contains 12 grams of carbohydrate. All forms of alcohol are empty calories providing no nutritional value. Diet beverages are sweetened with zero-calorie sweeteners that are anti-ketogenic. Black tea, coffee, and colas contain caffeine, which is a drug—a stimulant. If you are trying to simulate the effects of fasting, then you would not want your metabolism altered by drugs of any type. These effects can change the action of ketones and how they interact with our genes. As a stimulant, caffeine produces just the opposite effect as fasting or a ketogenic diet, which are calming, allowing the body to break down tissue, cleanse, and detoxify. Caffeine, in contrast, stimulates activity, growth, and accumulation.

During the ketogenic diet, thirst as well as hunger is usually blunted. Consequently, people often do not drink enough water during the day and become mildly dehydrated. Dehydration promotes kidney stone formation, causes constipation, promotes muscle cramps, and saps energy. You need to make sure you consume at least 6 to 8 cups (1.5 to 2 L) of water daily to avoid these side effects.

Myth 15: Fiber Needs to be Counted in Your Daily Carbohydrate Allotment

Dietary fiber is a carbohydrate. Total carbohydrate listed on food labels includes both fiber and net carbohydrate. Net carbohydrate is converted into glucose and raises blood sugar levels. Fiber is not broken down into glucose in humans because we do not possess the enzymes for this to happen. For this reason, it provides no calories and does not affect blood sugar levels.

Some people, however, claim that fiber is partially digested in the intestinal tract by gut bacteria and in this process glucose is released and absorbed into the bloodstream so that it does contribute some calories and affect blood sugar. Therefore, all sources of carbohydrate need to be included in your daily total allotment. This is simply not true.

It is true, however, that some bacteria can digest some types of fiber. In this process the glucose that is released is consumed immediately by the bacteria and is not absorbed into the bloodstream. In this process, fiber is converted into short chain fatty acids, which are absorbed by the cells lining the colon and used by them as a source of energy. Short chain fatty acids are fats, not carbohydrate. In a sense, fiber can provide some energy but the energy comes from fat, which is what you want with a ketogenic diet. Therefore, there is no need to count fiber as part of your carbohydrate allotment.

Myth 16: The Ketogenic Diet Makes You Weak and Lethargic

A common side effect when beginning the ketogenic diet is a lack of energy or endurance. The reason for this is that the body must transition from a metabolic state of burning glucose for energy to burning primarily fat. It takes some time for the body to make this adaptation. If your lifestyle is fairly sedentary, you may not notice any difference in your energy levels. It is most noticeable for active people, especially those who exercise regularly. If you are physically active, you will tire more quickly than usual or won't have the same level of endurance you normally do. Physical strength, however, is unaffected. If you were able to lift a 200-pound (90 kg) weight, you will still be able to do it, but you will tire sooner. This effect generally lasts between 1 to 2 weeks. Once your body has learned to burn fats efficiently, your normal energy levels will return. In time, you may even notice an increase in your endurance levels because you get more energy from fat than glucose and you have far more energy available to you from stored body fat than you ever could from stored glucose.

Once you have become keto adapted, your body will be primed to move more quickly and easily into ketosis the next time. When you go into ketosis, the period of time you feel fatigued will be shorter and may only last a few days.

Myth 17: The Ketogenic Diet Depresses Thyroid Function

Some people have claimed that going on a ketogenic diet depresses thyroid function. This will only happen if the diet is unbalanced and contains too much keto junk food, sugar substitutes, or polyunsaturated oils. A proper ketogenic diet, which is based around healthy low-carb vegetables supplemented with fresh meat, dairy, eggs, and occasional low-carb fruits along with good fats, will actually improve thyroid function.

The combination of excessive stress and a chronically undernourished diet can lead to low thyroid function. In fact, this is the primary cause of hypothyroidism. We live in a stressful world with worries and demands associated with education, career, job performance, personal and family relationships, congested traffic, illness, social and political distress, exposure to environmental and industrial toxins, and even the stress associated with pregnancy and childbirth. Consequently, many of us are in a continual state of stress.

When we are stressed, our body's demands for good nutrition are increased as essential vitamins and minerals are consumed at a high rate, so good nutrition is vitally important. Unfortunately, most people do not eat nutritionally dense foods, relying on ultra-processed, ready-to-eat or heat-and-serve convenience foods. Such foods are so highly processed that much of their original nutrition has been stripped away, leaving mostly empty calories. Consequently, we become subclinically malnourished. We consume just enough nutrients in our foods to keep from developing obvious nutritional deficiencies such as scurvy or beriberi, but not enough to maintain good health.

Subclinical malnutrition is intensified whenever a person goes on a low-fat, calorie restricted diet. Restricting calories and eliminating nourishing fats promotes poor nutrition. Whenever calorie intake is restricted enough to cause weight loss, the body instinctively interprets this as a famine. In order to reserve vital nutrients and survive the famine, thyroid function slows down. This is normal and natural. When refeeding resumes, the body senses the famine is over and thyroid function returns to normal. However, if the body is nutritionally bankrupt and refeeding involves nutritionally poor foods, the thyroid cannot recover properly and remains depressed.

After a low-fat, calorie-restricted diet, thyroid function can be stuck in low gear, leading to rapid weight gain. This is often followed by another low-fat, low-calorie diet which further lowers nutritional status and depresses thyroid function. Again, if the person ends the diet by eating the same high-carb, ultra-processed, low-nutrient foods, weight will rebound. This is often again followed by another attempt at dieting with the same result. Instead of losing weight through the course of these diets, more weight seems to accumulate after each one. In order to maintain the weight loss you must remain on a reduced calorie diet indefinitely, which will keep your thyroid in a perpetual state of depression.

Saturated fats have been villainized for so many years that people tend to shy away from them even when they go on a ketogenic diet, preferring to use vegetable oils in place of animal fats or tropical oils. This is a huge mistake. The ketogenic diet encourages the use of fat. However, excessive use of vegetable oil (more than about 10 percent of daily calories) can in itself depress thyroid function. Consuming polyunsaturated vegetable oils drains vital nutrients from the body. Polyunsaturated oils are highly vulnerable to oxidation and degradation. During this process highly reactive molecular enmities are formed called free radicals. These renegade molecules damage cells and tissues, including the mitochondria—the energy producing organelles in the cells, including thyroid cells. Our antioxidant defenses, which include vitamins A, C, D, E and nutrients such as beta-carotene, lycopene, and lutein, come to our defense by neutralizing these destructive molecules. However, in the process, these nutrients are destroyed, thus depleting these vital nutrients. These nutrients are not only involved in our defense against free radicals but are used for many other important functions in the body, so a deficiency can lead to poor health and depress thyroid function.

One of the benefits of using coconut oil is that it helps prevent the destructive action of free radicals and stimulates metabolism and thyroid function. The unique medium chain fatty acids in coconut oil boost metabolism of the body, this also boosts thyroid function. When combined with proper nutrition, the metabolic boosting effect of coconut oil can stimulate the thyroid to start working more efficiently.[5] Thus, a nutrient dense ketogenic diet, rich in coconut oil and low in polyunsaturated vegetables oils will support healthy thyroid function.

Myth 18: It Is Unhealthy to Eliminate Most or All Carbohydrate from the Diet

The ketogenic diet has been criticized as unhealthy because it strictly limits carbohydrate consumption. Critics claim we must have carbohydrate-rich foods in our diet because these types of foods provide important vitamins, minerals, and dietary fiber that are necessary for good health.

What most critics fail to understand is that the ketogenic diet does not eliminate all sources of carbohydrate. It is not an all meat and fat diet as some believe. Plant foods are an important part of the ketogenic diet. Net carbohydrate is limited to less than 50 grams per day. Starch and sugar are the biggest sources of carbohydrate in our diet. Eating foods containing large amounts of starch and sugar such as grains, starchy vegetables, and sweet fruits can easily surpass this limit, and therefore, are generally eliminated from the diet. However, low-carb vegetables, fruits, and nuts are an essential part of the ketogenic diet, and a healthy ketogenic diet should be centered around low-carb vegetables, supplemented by low-carb fruits, nuts, meat, fish, dairy, and eggs, and of course, healthy fats. These types of foods provide all of the vitamins, minerals, fiber, and other nutrients necessary for good health. In fact, because the standard diet most people eat is overloaded with processed grains, starchy vegetables, and sweets, all of which are nutrient poor, the ketogenic diet is generally far more nutrient-packed and generally the most nutritious diet most people have ever eaten in their lives.

Although the ketogenic diet does not focus on eating large amounts of meat, even an all meat and fat diet can provide adequate nutrients to sustain good health, as evidenced by the many meat-eating populations that have existed throughout history.

Myth 19: The Ketogenic Diet Is Nutritionally Unbalanced and Must Include Multiple Vitamin and Mineral Supplements to Prevent Deficiencies

At first glance, because many foods are restricted, including some healthy high-carb foods, it may seem that the ketogenic diet could be lacking in nutrients. That is not the case. This diet supplies all the nutrition a person needs to be healthy.

The diet should include plenty of fresh vegetables, both raw and cooked. You will be eating more vegetables than you probably have in your entire life. You could even call this a vegetable-based diet supplemented with ample fat and adequate protein. Fat enhances the absorption of the vitamins and minerals in foods. Simply adding fat to your meals increases the amount of nutrients you absorb from your food. The combination of healthy fats with fresh vegetables makes the ketogenic diet highly nutritious. A person can live a long and healthy life without eating grains, starchy vegetables, fruits, desserts and sweets, or ultra-processed foods. In fact, the diet is generally far healthier without most of these types of foods.

You certainly can add vitamin and mineral supplements if you wish, as there is no harm in it and in some cases supplementation can be helpful. High-carb diets tend to retain salt and electrolytes, like potassium and magnesium. It is known that both water fasting and ketogenic dieting lead to an accelerated water, sodium, and magnesium excretion through the urine. Therefore, you may want to increase your intake of sodium, magnesium, and potassium. You can tell if you need to increase your intake of these minerals if you experience muscle cramps. Add sodium by increasing your salt intake and using sea salt liberally on your foods. You can get additional magnesium (300 to 500 mg/day) and potassium (100 to 300 mg/day) from dietary supplements, from foods rich in these substances, or a combination of both.

Low-carb foods rich in magnesium in order of content include the following: spinach, shrimp, beet greens, broccoli, beets, oysters, zucchini, asparagus, seaweed, turnip greens, green beans, chicken, and beef. Low-carb foods rich in potassium in order include the following: spinach, bok choy, asparagus, beets, tomatoes, zucchini, broccoli, cauliflower, green beans, beef, parsley, and mushrooms.

Myth 20: People Diagnosed with Heart Disease, Diabetes, Cancer, or Some Other Serious Disease Should Not Attempt the Ketogenic Diet

Some people claim that if you have a serious health problem such as heart disease or diabetes, you should not go on a ketogenic diet. I have not seen any credible evidence to justify this precaution. Ironically, these are the very types of conditions that respond very well to the ketogenic diet and keto cycling. In fact, the ketogenic diet is potentially the most effective and least harmful treatment currently available for these conditions.

Excessive intake of carbohydrate, especially in the form of sugar and refined starch, is known to promote and exacerbate these conditions. Reducing carbohydrate intake has proven to highly effective in reducing their severity. The ketogenic diet is not harmful in any way and provides a good way to reduce refined carbohydrate intake. Keto cycling promotes autophagy to removed damaged and diseased cells, including arterial plaque and cancer cells, and stimulates rebuilding and repair with new, healthy stem cells. It makes sense to take advantage of the body's own power of cleansing and healing to overcome these conditions.

Myth 21: The Ketogenic Diet Will Adversely Affect Your Gut Microbiome

Your gut microbiome is the community of microorganisms living in your digestive tract. Most of these microbes are beneficial. They help digest our food, condition and train our immune system, regulate carbohydrate metabolism, produce important vitamins such as B_{12} and K, and prevent proliferation of unhealthy microbes, among other benefits.

Whenever you make a change to your diet—reduce calorie consumption, change the types of foods eaten, and even make only slight changes—your gut microbiome changes in response. Some foods, such as sugar and refined starch, encourage the proliferation of undesirable microbes and alter the gut microbiome in unhealthy ways.

Going on a ketogenic diet will change the percentages of the types of microorganisms that inhabit your gut. This change isn't necessarily bad or harmful. It is just a change to best facilitate and process the types of foods eaten. Consequently, bowel habits may change as well. This is normal and natural.

Myth 22: The Ketogenic Diet Causes Constipation and Diarrhea

Some people complain of diarrhea when they go keto. The reason for this is that the body has not fully adjusted to processing all the fat in the diet. Over the past several decades, fat has been shunned, and people have been eating low-fat and nonfat foods for so long that their bodies are not accustomed to digesting the amount of fat in the ketogenic diet. It takes time to adapt. Eating an adequate amount of high-fiber, low-carb foods (i.e. vegetables and nuts) can help reduce stomach discomfort and diarrhea from eating high amounts of fat.

In contrast, some people experience the opposite effect and have a hard time eliminating. On the ketogenic diet people generally eat less food than they normally do, so there will naturally be less to eliminate. Don't assume the lack of a need to empty the bowels is a sign of constipation. However, some people truly are constipated. One of the main reasons for this is dehydration. Keto dieters often don't feel the need to drink, and consequently don't drink enough and become dehydrated. You need to make sure you drink plenty of water throughout the day. Some people go almost all day without a drink of water; don't do that. Drink at least 6 to 8 cups (1.5 to 2 L) of water daily.

Constipation could also be caused by eating too much meat and not enough high-fiber vegetables or fat. The fiber in the vegetables will help with digestive function and elimination. Large quantities of fat also tend to loosen the bowels. If these changes do not work, you can loosen the bowels by taking a 250 to 300 mg magnesium supplement daily. You can also take 2,000 to 5,000 mg of vitamin C if the magnesium supplement alone does not work satisfactorily.

Myth 23: The Ketogenic Diet Is Only Good for Weight Loss

Most of the popularity surrounding the ketogenic diet is centered on its weight loss effects, but it is far more than just an effective slimming diet. It can improve mental function, blood sugar control, and cardiovascular health, protect against cancer, and stop chronic disease. Nearly all of the health markers that doctors measure to evaluate a patient's health are improved with a ketogenic diet.

The ketogenic diet can help you with the following:

- Reduce blood glucose and improve insulin sensitivity
- Reduce blood insulin levels
- Raise HDL cholesterol
- Reduce blood triglycerides
- Increase large, beneficial LDL cholesterol
- Reduce small, dense, potentially harmful cholesterol
- Reduce body weight and body mass index (BMI)
- Reduce waist circumference (reduce abdominal or visceral fat)
- Normalize blood pressure
- Reduce cholesterol ratio (total cholesterol/HDL)
- Reduce triglyceride ratio (triglyceride/HDL)
- Reduce C-reactive protein (a marker for systemic inflammation)
- Increase human growth hormone (HGH) levels
- Reduce advanced glycation end products (AGEs)
- Reduce free radicals and oxidative stress
- Improve mental function

The ketogenic diet improves the markers that are associated with elevated risk of heart attacks, strokes, diabetes, Alzheimer's, and other degenerative diseases, as well as reducing the processes that promote aging, thus preserving good health and extending healthspan (healthy lifespan).

For decades researchers have studied the life-extending effects of calorie restricted diets, wherein total daily calorie intake is reduced by 20 to 40 percent. In animals, lifespan has increased by as much as 40 percent simply by reducing the amount of food they eat. A recent study suggests that a ketogenic diet could increase healthspan by as much as 10 years. In the study adult mice were assigned to one of three diets: a ketogenic, low-carb, or control diet. As the mice aged, only those on the ketogenic diet maintained their youthful physiological function. These mice consuming the high-fat ketogenic diet saw a 13 percent increase in lifespan over the other two diets, which would translate into 10 extra years in humans.[6]

Myth 24: Ketone Dietary Supplements Are as Effective as the Ketogenic Diet

Many of the benefits associated with the ketogenic diet came from the body's use of ketones as a major source of fuel. Ketones are a much more efficient source of energy than glucose and activate certain genes associated with improved health and protection from disease. Studies have shown that ketones themselves can produce many desirable effects including the following:

Appetite suppression and weight loss
Improved cognition/memory
Increased energy
Better mood
Increased endurance and athletic performance
Reduced inflammation
Better sleep

Traditionally, the only way you could increase blood ketone levels was by going on a ketogenic diet, fasting, or by consuming a source of medium chain fatty acids, such as coconut or MCT oil. In recent years, ketone dietary supplements have entered the market. These are not MCTs but ketone salts that directly raise blood levels of the ketone beta-hydroxybutyrate or BHB. Ketone salts are made of BHB that are combined with potassium, calcium, sodium, or magnesium to improve absorption. This is the type of ketone currently used in all commercial dietary supplements. Researchers use another form, called ketone esters, in which BHB is linked to an alcohol, but they are very expensive and currently only used in research. These products are referred to as *exogenous* ketones because they originate from a source outside the body. This is in contrast to *endogenous* ketones, which are produced in the body by the liver.

The advantage of supplemental ketones is that they provide an almost instant source of ketones without the need to change the diet or consume large quantities of MCT oil or coconut oil. Exogenous ketones provide all the same health benefits that you get from the ketones produced when you go on a keto diet. For many people, it is far easier to stir a spoonful of ketones into a glass of water or juice and drink it than it is to make dramatic changes to the diet or take several spoonfuls of MCT oil. Another benefit is that it is less likely to upset the stomach like large amounts of MCT oil or coconut oil can. With exogenous ketones you can raise blood ketones to therapeutic levels with one dose mixed with a little water. Exogenous ketone supplements will raise blood ketones for about 2 to 3 hours and can be taken up to three times a day.

There are also some disadvantages to exogenous ketones. The most noticeable is the terrible taste. Some brands add flavorings and sweeteners to their products to make them more palatable. Sometimes people forget that these are dietary supplements, not shakes or beverages, and they aren't supposed to taste like candy.

Another issue is the price. The process of making ketone salts is expensive and for this reason, exogenous ketones supplements are pricey. You will pay $40 to $60 for one container that may provide 16 to 20 servings. In general, you would expect to pay anywhere from $2 to $4 per serving. The more expensive brands cost as much as $6.50 per serving. Companies often recommend two servings at day. This means 60 servings per month for a total of $390 monthly. That's a lot to pay for a supplement.

One of the other major disadvantages of using exogenous ketone supplements is that doing so does not effectively reduce blood glucose levels or reverse insulin resistance. If ketone supplements are used in place of going on a ketogenic diet, carbohydrate intake is not reduced. You do not benefit from the reduction in blood glucose levels. Your body remains in glucosis, burning glucose as its primary source of fuel. Ketones are used as well, but the body does not shift into a state of fat burning. Body fat is not pulled out of storage and burned. Although blood ketones can rise to measurable levels, you are not in a true state of ketosis. The metabolic switch from glucosis to ketosis does not occur. Genes that are activated or deactivated by the switch from glucosis to ketosis and back again remain unchanged.

Since total calorie intake is not reduced, the body does not go into autophagy, removing old and damaged tissues, nor does it come out of autophagy, which triggers the development of stem cells and growth of new, healthy tissues. Degenerative or damaged insulin-producing beta cells in the pancreas are not removed and replaced, so diabetes continues. Cancer, which feeds on sugar, can still survive on the carbohydrates and sugar consumed. With epilepsy, even when blood ketones are high, the addition of carbohydrate into the diet can initiate seizures. Excessive body fat is not utilized for energy, so there is no weight reduction or fat loss.

Taking an exogenous ketone supplement is much like taking any other dietary supplement; it can have some benefit, but it is definitely not a replacement for a good diet, or in this case, a ketogenic diet. If you want to take advantage of all of the health benefits offered by a ketogenic diet and keto cycling, you need to make dietary changes which involve reducing both total calorie and carbohydrate intake.

9

Fasting Mimicking Diet Recipes

The fasting mimicking diet (FMD) is a low-carb, low-protein, low-calorie, ketogenic diet. It is a modified fast that allows a minimal amount of nutrients. For best results, the total daily calorie intake should be limited to 600 or less. At this level the body is still undernourished, much like a water fast, but provides just enough nutrition to enhance the cleansing and healing process. Allowing a single small meal also makes the fast a little more tolerable than a strict water fast and provides enough energy to maintain normal day-to-day activities including moderate exercise if that is a part of your normal routine.

It is important that you do the fast correctly in order to fully activate autophagy. This is why you must restrict carbohydrate and protein as well as calories. Salads are the most suitable meals for this type of diet. Meal planning is easy, a simple tossed salad using a variety of low-carb vegetables is all you need.

Other options are stir fries and soups. Salads are generally preferred because it takes longer to chew and eat raw vegetables, providing more time to enjoy the meal. Also, raw vegetables take a little longer to digest so you can feel satisfied longer. However, after eating salads every day, sometimes it is nice to have a break and eat something different. Sample FMD salad, stir fry, and soup recipes are provided in the following pages.

FMD TOSSED SALAD

A variety of suitable salads can be made without the hassle of looking up the specifics of every ingredient and trying to calculate the grams of net carbohydrate, protein, and fat every time you make a meal. Simply follow the formula below and keep track of the total calories as described.

3 cups (27 g) leafy greens, cut into bite-size pieces (see list below)
2 cups (50 g) low-carb salad vegetables, cut into bite-size pieces (see list below)
½ avocado, sliced (optional)
3-6 tablespoons (45-90 ml) salad dressing

Combine the leafy greens and low-carb vegetables into a serving bowl. Select your vegetables from the two lists below. Add avocado if desired. Top with a salad dressing of your choice (choices listed below).

This recipe serves one person. Double the recipe for two people. Without salad dressing or avocado each serving contains about 77 calories; with half an avocado total calories increase to 217. For the final calorie count, add the salad dressing calories indicated with each dressing recipe. For example, 3 tablespoons of the Oil and Vinegar Dressing adds 150 calories for a total of 367 calories.

Leafy Greens
Lettuce (any variety)
Cabbage
Spinach
Chinese cabbage
Kale
Parsley
Cilantro
Water cress

Each cup (60 g) of mixed leafy greens contains on average about 9 calories.

143

Low-Carb Salad Vegetables
Bamboo shoots
Bell peppers
Broccoli
Carrot
Cauliflower
Celeriac (celery root)
Celery
Cucumber
Daikon radish
Fennel
Green beans (pickled or cooked)
Olives
Radish
Sauerkraut
Scallions
Sprouts (alfalfa, clover, broccoli, radish)
Tomato
Turnip
Water chestnuts
Zucchini

Each cup (108 g) of mixed low-carb vegetables contains on average about 25 calories.

Optional Ingredients

Avocado is a great addition to salads because it increases the total fat content and adds flavor. One average-size Hass avocado contains about 280 calories, and half an avocado contains roughly 140 calories.

If you have room for additional calories you may also include a *small* portion of low-carb nuts. Suitable nuts include almonds, pecans, macadamia, Brazil, hazelnut, walnut, and coconut. One-fourth cup (28g) of these nuts contains on average about 190 calories, so you can't use too much. Do not use any other type of nut or seed as they have a much higher carb content.

You may also add a small amount of shredded cheese, such as parmesan or cheddar. One tablespoon (5 g) of shredded cheese has 20 calories and 2 grams of protein. If you use cheese limit yourself to 4 tablespoons (20 g) or less, as otherwise you will be adding too much protein.

You can adjust the quantity of salad ingredients in any way you desire with the goal of staying under 600 total calories. By changing the types of vegetables and the salad dressings you use, you can eat a different salad every day.

Salad Dressings

You should avoid all commercially prepared salad dressings, even the so-called organic or natural dressings. They all contain ingredients you don't want in your diet, such as sugar, artificial sweeteners, flavor enhancers, preservatives, dyes, and emulsifiers, canola or soybean oils, and other undesirable vegetable oils.

Below are 4 salad dressings you can make at home that are suitable. Simply combine and mix the ingredients to make each dressing.

Olive Oil and Herbs
3 tablespoons (15 ml) extra virgin olive oil
¼ teaspoon Italian herbs
Salt and pepper to taste

Makes 3 tablespoons; 126 calories per tablespoon (15 ml).

Oil and Vinegar Dressing
¼ cup (60 ml) extra virgin olive oil
¼ cup (60 ml) apple cider vinegar
2 tablespoons (30 ml) water
Dash salt and pepper

Makes 10 tablespoons (90 g); 50 calories per tablespoon (15 ml).

Thousand Island Dressing
2 tablespoons (28 g) mayonnaise*
1 tablespoon (14 g) low-sugar catsup
2 teaspoons dill pickle relish

¼ teaspoon onion power
Dash salt and pepper

*Use a brand of mayonnaise made with avocado, olive, or coconut oils. Avoid mayonnaise made with canola and soybean oils.

Makes about 3½ tablespoons (49 g); 63 calories per tablespoon (14 g).

Ranch Dressing
3 tablespoons (28 g) full-fat sour cream
1 tablespoon (15 ml) cream or milk
¼ teaspoon onion powder
Dash salt and pepper

Makes 4 tablespoons (60 ml); 33 calories per tablespoon (15 ml).

STIR FRY AND SOUP RECIPES
Use any mix of vegetables in the list below for stir frying and soups. You can use any type of herb or spice in addition to these, but avoid any commercial herb or spice mixes that contain sugar or questionable ingredients. Use any one or more of the fats listed below for cooking.

Low-Carb Vegetables for Cooking
Asparagus
Bamboo shoots
Bean sprouts (mung)
Bell peppers
Broccoli
Cabbage
Chinese cabbage
Carrot
Cauliflower
Celery
Chard

Eggplant
Garlic
Green beans
Leeks
Mushrooms
Onion
Spinach
Yellow neck squash
Zucchini

Each cup (94 g) of mixed vegetables contains on average about 20 calories.

Fats and Oils for Cooking
Bacon drippings
Beef tallow
Butter
Coconut oil
Extra virgin olive oil
Ghee
Lard
Red palm oil

Most fats and oils contain 126 calories per tablespoon. Coconut oil contains 120 and butter 110 calories per tablespoon (14 g).

Vegetable Stir Fry
This stir fry recipe allows 1 slice of bacon for flavoring if desired. A single slice of bacon is mostly fat and provides only 3 grams of protein. The best oils for moderate to high temperature cooking are lard, beef tallow, coconut oil, red palm oil, and ghee. For low to moderate cooking you can use butter or extra virgin olive oil.

1 medium slice sugar-free bacon, chopped (optional)
2 tablespoons (30 ml) oil
3 cups (282 g) low-carb vegetables for cooking, cut into bite-size pieces

Heat a skillet to moderate heat. Cut bacon into several pieces and put into the skillet as it is heating up. Add oil and vegetables and sauté until done. Add salt, pepper, and herbs to taste.

An optional ingredient is soy sauce. One tablespoon (15 ml) contains 10 calories and 2 grams of protein.

Makes one serving; total calorie count without oil or soy sauce is 106. With 2 tablespoons (30 ml) of oil and 1 tablespoon (15 ml) soy sauce total calorie count is 368. You can add another 1 or 2 cups of vegetables if you like and still remain under 600 calories.

Vegetable Soup

You can use chicken, beef, or vegetable broth in this recipe. One cup of commercially produced chicken or beef broth contains 4 calories and 3 grams of protein. Use any mixture you like of the low-carb vegetables for cooking listed above. Chicken broth and butter provide a rich flavor, which can be supplemented by the addition of any herbs or spices you would like to add.

1½ cups (360 ml) broth
2 cups mixture of onions, mushrooms, carrots, and celery,
    cut into bite-size pieces*
2 tablespoons (28 g) butter or oil of your choice
¼ teaspoon onion powder
Herbs and spices (as desired)**
2 tablespoons (10 g) shredded parmesan cheese (optional)
Salt and pepper to taste

Pour broth into a small cooking pot and heat to boiling. Add vegetables, butter, onion power, and herbs; reduce heat and simmer for about 10 minutes or until vegetables are tender. Remove from heat and stir in cheese, salt, and pepper. Serve.

* You can use any combination of vegetables from the low-carb vegetables for cooking.

**Some possible suggestions include garlic, sage, rosemary, thyme, marjoram, curry powder, ginger, coriander, and garam masala.

An optional ingredient is tomato paste. One tablespoon (15 g) of tomato paste contains 15 calories and 3.5 grams of carbs. Because it has a fairly high amount of carbs, you don't want to use too much. For this recipe you can add up to 2 tablespoons of tomato paste. This makes a tomato vegetable soup.

Makes about 3 cups (700 ml); total calorie count without tomato paste is 316, with 2 tablespoons of tomato paste calorie count increases to 346.

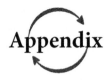

Appendix

Keto Bookshelf

DR. FIFE'S KETO COOKERY
Nutritious and Delicious Ketogenic Recipes
for Healthy Living
By Bruce Fife, ND

Many of the so-called ketogenic recipes found online and in cookbooks are not actually ketogenic. Simply because a recipe may be low-carb does not make it ketogenic or keto friendly. Ironically, many of these recipes contain ingredients that make them anti-ketogenic and incompatible with a ketogenic diet. The vast majority of ketogenic cookbooks on the market today contain many recipes that are not ketogenic. Using such sources can sabotage your efforts to reach ketosis and gain the benefits of the ketogenic diet and keto cycling.

For this reason, Dr. Bruce Fife has compiled into one volume his favorite ketogenic recipes. Described as the ultimate ketogenic cookbook, it contains nearly 450 recipes, including 70 vegetable recipes, 47 salads and 22 dressings, 60 egg recipes, 50 delicious high-fat sauces for meats and vegetables, as well as a variety of mouthwatering wraps, soups, and casseroles, with a creative array of meat, fish, and poultry dishes. With this resource, you will always have plenty of options to choose from for your daily needs.

No exotic or hard-to-find ingredients here. This is a practical cookbook that can be used every day for life. All of the recipes are simple, with ingredients that are readily available at your local grocery store. None of the recipes include any artificial sweeteners, sugars, flavor enhancers, gluten, grains, or other questionable ingredients. Recipes use only fresh, wholesome, natural foods to guarantee optimal health.

Examples of some of the recipes in this book include: chicken pot pie, corned beef and cabbage, barbecue beef short ribs, sirloin tip roast with roasted vegetables, roasted rolled pork belly with mushroom stuffing, rosemary lemon pork chops, lamb patties with mushroom gravy, shepherd's pie, low-carb turkey dressing, crispy chicken wings, Parmesan chicken strips, pecan-breaded fish fillets, breakfast pizza, coco fries, avocado bacon wraps, and beef stroganoff.

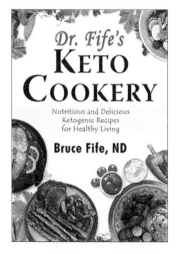

Dr. Fife's Keto Cookery is available from the publisher at www. piccadillybooks.com or from Amazon at https://goo.gl/WrZgea.

THE COCONUT KETOGENIC DIET
Supercharge Your Metabolism, Revitalize Thyroid Function, and Lose Excess Weight
By Bruce Fife, ND

You can enjoy eating rich, full-fat foods and lose weight without counting calories or suffering from hunger. The secret is a high-fat, ketogenic diet. Our bodies need fat. It's necessary for optimal health. It's also necessary in order to lose weight safely and naturally.

Low-fat diets have been heavily promoted for the past three decades, and as a result we are fatter now than ever before. Obviously, there is something wrong with the low-fat approach to weight loss. This book exposes many common myths and misconceptions about fats and weight loss and explains why low-fat diets don't work. It also reveals new, cutting-edge research on one of the world's most exciting weight loss aids—coconut oil—and how you can use it to power up your metabolism, boost your energy, improve thyroid function, and lose unwanted weight.

This revolutionary weight loss program is designed to keep you both slim and healthy using wholesome, natural foods, and the most health-promoting fats. It has proven successful in helping those suffering from obesity, diabetes, heart and circulatory problems, low thyroid function, chronic fatigue, high blood pressure, high cholesterol, and many other conditions.

In this book you will learn: why you need to eat fat to lose fat; why you should not eat lean protein without a source of fat; how to lose weight without feeling hungry or miserable; how to stop food cravings dead cold; how to use your diet to overcome common health problems; how to reach your ideal weight and stay there; why eating rich, delicious foods can help you lose weight; and which foods are the real troublemakers and how to avoid them.

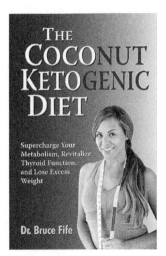

The Coconut Ketogenic Diets is available from the publisher at www. piccadillybooks.com or from Amazon at https://goo.gl/cquUCV.

KETONE THERAPY
The Ketogenic Cleanse and Anti-Aging Diet
By Bruce Fife, ND

The ketogenic diet is one that is very low in carbohydrate, high in fat, with moderate protein. This diet shifts the body into a natural, healthy metabolic state known as nutritional ketosis.

In ketosis the body uses fat as its primary source of energy instead of glucose. Some of this fat is converted into an alternative form of fuel called ketones. Ketones are high-potency fuel that boost energy and cellular efficiency and activates special enzymes that regulate cell survival, repair, and growth. When a person is in nutritional ketosis, blood levels of ketones are elevated to therapeutic levels. In response, high blood pressure drops, cholesterol levels improve, inflammation is reduced, blood sugar levels normalize, and overall health improves.

Low-fat diets have been heavily promoted for the past several decades as the answer to obesity and chronic disease. However, we are fatter and sicker now more than ever before. Obviously, the low-fat approach has not worked. Our bodies actually need fat for optimal health and function more efficiently using fat for fuel.

In this book, you will discover how people are successfully using the ketogenic diet to prevent and treat chronic and degenerative disease. Ketone therapy is backed by decades of medical and clinical research, which has proven the method to be both safe and effective for the treatment of variety of health issues. Topics covered include

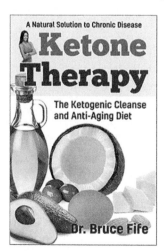

neurodegenerative disorders, neurodevelopmental disorders, diabetes and metabolic syndrome, detoxification and immune function, digestive disorders, cancer, and much more.

Many health problems that medical science has deemed incurable or untreatable are being reversed. Medications that were once relied on daily are no longer necessary and are being tossed away. People are discovering that a simple, but revolutionary diet based on wholesome, natural foods and the most health-promoting fats is dramatically changing their lives.

Ketone Therapy is available from the publisher at www. piccadillybooks.com or from Amazon at https://goo.gl/A7NrhM.

STOP ALZHEIMER'S NOW!
How to Prevent and Reverse Dementia, Parkinson's, ALS, Multiple Sclerosis, and Other Neurodegenerative Disorders
By Bruce Fife, ND
Foreword by Russell L. Blaylock, MD

More than 35 million people have dementia today. Alzheimer's disease is the most common form of dementia. Millions more suffer with other neurodegenerative disorders. The number of people affected by these destructive diseases continues to increase every year.

The brain is fully capable of functioning normally for a lifetime, regardless of how long a person lives. While aging is a risk factor for neurodegeneration, it is not the cause! Dementia and other neurodegenerative disorders are disease processes that can be prevented and successfully treated.

This book outlines a program using ketone therapy and diet that is backed by decades of medical and clinical research and has proven successful in restoring mental function and improving both brain and overall health. You will learn how to prevent and even reverse symptoms associated with Alzheimer's disease, Parkinson's disease, amyotrophic lateral sclerosis (ALS), multiple sclerosis (MS), Huntington's disease, epilepsy, diabetes, stroke, and various forms of dementia.

The information in this book is also useful for anyone who wants to be spared from encountering these devastating afflictions. These diseases don't happen overnight. They take years, often decades, to develop.

You *can* stop Alzheimer's and other neurodegenerative diseases now before they take over your life.

"A must read for everyone concerned with Alzheimer's disease... the author explains how diet modifications and the addition of coconut oil can drastically change the course of the disease."
Edmond Devroey, MD
The Longevity Institute

"*Stop Alzheimer's Now!*...will not only be beneficial for Alzheimer's but also for a wide variety of other diseases. I strongly recommend reading this book!"
Sofie Hexebert, MD, PhD

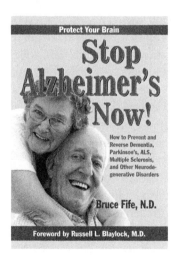

Stop Alzheimer's Now! is available from the publisher at www. piccadillybooks.com or from Amazon at https://goo.gl/2t44Ez.

STOP VISION LOSS NOW!
Prevent and Heal Cataracts, Glaucoma, Macular Degeneration, and Other Common Eye Disorders
By Bruce Fife, ND

Losing your eyesight is a frightening thought. Yet, every five seconds someone in the world goes blind. Most causes of visual impairment are caused by age-related diseases such as cataracts, glaucoma, macular degeneration, and diabetic retinopathy. Modern medicine has no cure for these conditions. Treatment usually involves managing the symptoms and attempting to slow the progression of the disease. In some cases surgery is an option, but there is always the danger of adverse side effects that can damage the eyes even further.

Most chronic progressive eye disorders are considered incurable, hopeless. However, there is a successful treatment. It doesn't involve surgery, drugs, or invasive medical procedures. All that is needed is a proper diet. The key is coconut, specifically coconut oil, combined with a low-carb or ketogenic diet. The author used this method to cure is own glaucoma, something standard medical therapy is unable to do.

The coconut based dietary program described in this book has the potential to help prevent and treat many common visual problems including the following: cataracts, glaucoma, macular degeneration, diabetic retinopathy, dry eye syndrome, Sjogren's syndrome, optic neuritis, irritated eyes, conjunctivitis (pink eye), and eye disorders related to neurodegenerative disease (Alzheimer's, Parkinson's, stroke, MS)

Most chronic eye disorders come without warning. No one can tell who will develop a visual handicap as they age. Everybody is at risk. Once the disease is present, treatment is a lifelong process. The best solution is prevention.

In this book, you will learn the basic underlying causes for the most common degenerative eye disorders and what you can do to prevent, stop, and even reverse them.

"Well-researched, comprehensive, and interesting. Dr. Fife has a gift for making advanced nutrition concepts and physiological processes easy for the average reader to understand...There are many personal accounts throughout the book, including the author's story of how he reversed his own early-stage glaucoma."

Franziska Spritzler, RD, CDE

"Skeptical that treating my eyes with the suggestions outlined in this book, I nevertheless began to do them. I have been virtually stunned that just after 2 weeks..the pain in both eyes is completely gone, the scratchy feelings, eye fatigue, and eye dryness are now a thing of the past...My recovery is real, and I have been able to return full time to using my computer."

Maria Atwood, *Wise Traditions*, Weston A. Price Foundation.

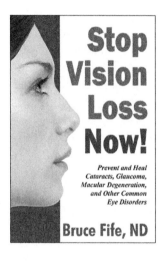

Stop Vision Loss Now! is available from the publisher at www. piccadillybooks.com or from Amazon at https://goo.gl/LbQYL9.

STOP AUTISM NOW!
A Parent's Guide to Preventing and Reversing Autism Spectrum Disorders
By Bruce Fife, ND

Over 1 million people have autism. This number is rapidly growing. Over the past several years autism has increased to epidemic proportions. Thirty years ago it affected only 1 in 2,500; today 1 out of every 50 children in the United States is affected.

Over the past 12 years there has been a 17 percent increase in childhood developmental disabilities of all types including autism, attention deficit hyperactivity disorder (ADHD), epilepsy, mental retardation, and others. Currently in the United States, 4 million children have ADHD, the most common learning disability, and an incredible one in six children are classified as learning disabled.

Why the sudden astronomical rise in developmental disabilities? Most doctors have no clue what causes autism, nor any idea how to prevent or treat it. The only medically recognized form of treatment is an attempt to teach affected children how to manage the disorder and live with it. Antidepressants, antipsychotics, and stimulants are often prescribed to help them cope with their symptoms. No possibility of a cure is offered, as the condition is considered hopeless.

Autism, however, is not a hopeless condition. It can be prevented and successfully treated without the use of drugs. This book describes an innovative new dietary and lifestyle approach involving coconut ketone therapy that has proven very successful in reversing even some of the most severe developmental disorders, allowing once disabled children to enter regular school and lead normal, happy, productive lives. There is a solution. You can stop autism now!

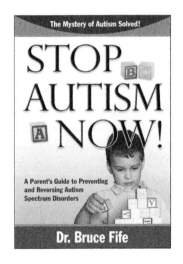

"Autism is a subject that I have spent a good deal of time analyzing, researching, and writing about and no one does a better job condensing and explaining what is known about this terrible disorder than does Doctor Fife. His advice, designed to treat this disorder, is based on good science and practical experience."

Russell L. Blaylock, MD
Board Certified Neurosurgeon
Author of *Excitotoxins: The Taste That Kills*

Stop Autism Now! is available from the publisher at www. piccadillybooks.com or from Amazon at https://goo.gl/Mk1urP.

FAT HEALS, SUGAR KILLS
The Cause of and Cure to Cardiovascular Disease, Diabetes, Obesity, and Other Metabolic Disorders
By Bruce Fife, ND

For decades we've been avoiding fat like the plague, eating low-fat this, non-fat that, choosing egg whites over the yokes, and trimming off every morsel of fat from meat in order to comply with the *US Dietary Guidelines* recommendation to reduce our fat intake.

As a whole, we have succeeded in reducing our total fat intake and replacing it with more so-called "healthy" carbohydrates—most notably refined grains and sugar. What has been the consequence? Obesity is at an all-time high, diabetes and metabolic disorders have increased to epidemic proportions. Heart disease is still our number one killer. We have dutifully followed the advice of the "experts" and as a result, we are sicker now more than ever before.

What went wrong? You can give thanks to the sugar industry. Through clever marketing, misdirection, flawed science, and powerful lobbying, the sugar industry succeeded in diverting attention away from themselves and putting the blame on fat, particularly saturated fat. We fell for it hook, line, and sinker.

Replacing fat with refined carbohydrates was the worse dietary blunder of the 20th century and has led to the skyrocketing levels of chronic disease we are experiencing today. Fortunately, there is a solution—cut out the refined carbohydrates and add good fats back into the diet. New research is showing that fats are essential nutrients with important functions and can be used to help prevent and even reverse heart disease, diabetes, cancer, Alzheimer's, and many other chronic degenerative diseases that are caused by or made worse by the overconsumption of refined carbohydrates.

This book explains how sugar and refined carbohydrates are destroying our health. It also reveals new evidence and cutting-edge science behind the incredible healing potential of dietary fats and explains how and why certain fats are now considered not only healthy, but some of our most powerful superfoods.

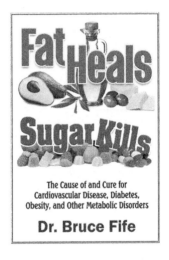

Fat Heals, Sugar Kills is available from the publisher at www.piccadillybooks.com or from Amazon at https://amzn.to/2WlCDqA.

THE STEVIA DECEPTION
The Hidden Dangers of Low-Calorie Sweeteners
By Bruce Fife, ND

Through the power of persuasive advertising and cleaver marketing we've been sold on the idea that stevia is a natural, herbal sweetener that is not only harmless but even health-promoting. As such, it is promoted as a better choice over sugar or other low-calorie sweeteners. Stevia has rapidly become a multimillion dollar industry.

Despite all of the marketing hype, stevia is not the innocent little herb it is made out to be and it is not harmless. The stevia sweetener you purchase at the store is a highly refined, purified chemical that is little different from any other artificial sweetener, with many of the same drawbacks and dangers. To say that stevia is harmless because it is derived from an herb, is like saying sugar or cocaine are harmless because they too are derived from herbs.

The author's observation of troubling adverse reactions associated with stevia led him on an investigation that revealed disturbing facts hidden from the public, including studies that contradict the sweetener's safety and assumed benefits.

In this book, you will learn why you should never use stevia if you want to lose excess weight or control diabetes. You will also learn why all low-calorie sweeteners are potentially dangerous and what options you have available. The information in this book comes directly from published studies, historical facts, and the author's own personal experiences.

"I am a kinesiologist (32 years). I test foods, supplements, etc. I've never found a stevia product that anyone tested positive on. I didn't know why [but after reading this book] now I do. Just like people think a lot of herbs and supplements are safe, yet I know by [kinesiology] testing that they are not."

Marene

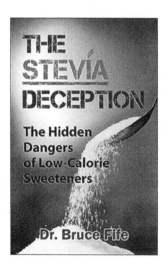

The Stevia Deception is available from the publisher at www.piccadillybooks.com or from Amazon at https://goo.gl/rMdhKM.

THE COCONUT OIL MIRACLE
5th Edition
By Bruce Fife, ND
Foreword by Jon J. Kabara, PhD

Dr. Fife was the first person to gather together all the medical research on coconut oil and present it in a readable and understandable format. This best-selling book describes the many health benefits of coconut oil and dispels the untruths surrounding this often misunderstood oil.

Benefits of Coconut Oil include:
• Reduces risk of atherosclerosis and heart disease
• Reduces risk of cancer and other degenerative conditions
• Helps prevent bacterial, viral, and fungal (including yeast) infections
• Supports immune system function
• Helps prevent osteoporosis
• Helps control diabetes
• Promotes weight loss
• Enhances ketogenesis
• Provides an immediate source of energy
• Improves digestion and nutrient absorption
• Has a mild delicate flavor
• Is highly resistant to spoilage (long shelf life)
• Is heat resistant (the healthiest oil for cooking)
• Helps keep skin soft and smooth
• Helps prevent premature aging and wrinkling of the skin
• Helps protect against skin cancer and other blemishes

Coconut oil has been called the healthiest dietary oil on earth. If you're not using coconut oil for your daily cooking and body care needs you're missing out on one of nature's most amazing health products.

"Dr. Bruce Fife should be commended for bringing together in this very readable book the positive health benefits of coconut oil. The inquiring reader will have a new and more balanced view of the role of fat and especially saturated fats in our diet."

Jon Kabara, PhD
Professor Emeritus,
Michigan State University

"He does a fabulous job of documenting how coconut oil, a saturated fat, is actually beneficial to your heart...Fife's book explains in great detail many of the other great healing aspects of this forgotten oil. I heartily recommend you get a copy of the book and study it for yourself."

William Campbell Douglass, MD
Second Opinion

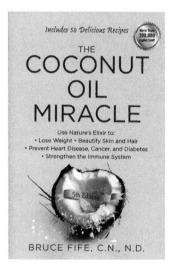

The Coconut Oil Miracle is available from the publisher at www. piccadillybooks.com or from Amazon at https://goo.gl/GYit3Y.

THE PALM OIL MIRACLE
By Bruce Fife, ND

Palm oil has been used as both a food and a medicine for thousands of years. It was prized by the pharaohs of ancient Egypt as a sacred food. Today palm oil is the most widely used oil in the world. In tropical Africa and Southeast Asia it is an integral part of a healthy diet just as olive oil is in the Mediterranean.

Palm oil possesses excellent cooking properties. It is more heat stable than other vegetable oils and imparts in foods and baked goods superior taste, texture, and quality.

Palm oil is one of the world's healthiest oils. As a natural vegetable oil, it contains no trans fatty acids or cholesterol. It is currently being used by doctors and government agencies to treat specific illnesses and improve nutritional status. Recent medical studies have shown that palm oil, particularly virgin (red) palm oil, can protect against many common health problems. Some of the health benefits include:

• Improves blood circulation
• Protects against heart disease
• Protects against cancer
• Boosts immunity
• Improves blood sugar control
• Improves nutrient absorption and vitamin and mineral status
• Aids in the prevention and treatment of malnutrition
• Supports healthy lung and liver function
• Helps strengthen bones and teeth
• Supports eye health
• Helps protect against mental deterioration, including Alzheimer's disease
• Richest dietary source of vitamin E and beta-carotene

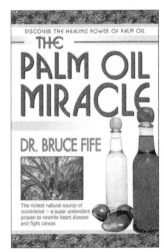

DISCOVER THE HEALING POWER OF PALM OIL

THE

PALM OIL MIRACLE

DR. BRUCE FIFE

The richest natural source of tocotrienol – a super antioxidant proven to reverse heart disease and fight cancer.

The Palm Oil Miracle is available from the publisher at www. piccadillybooks.com or from Amazon at https://goo.gl/zMVGTi.

COCONUT CURES
Preventing and Treating Common Health Problems with Coconut
By Bruce Fife, ND
Foreword by Conrado S. Dayrit, MD

Discover the amazing health benefits of coconut oil, meat, milk, and water. In this book you will learn why coconut oil is considered the healthiest oil on earth and how it can protect you against heart disease, diabetes, and infectious illnesses such as influenza, herpes, Candida, and even HIV.

There is more to the healing power of coconut than just the oil. You will also learn about the amazing health benefits of coconut meat, milk, and water. You will learn why coconut water is used as an IV solution and how coconut meat can protect you from colon cancer, regulate blood sugar, and expel intestinal parasites. Contains dozens of fascinating case studies and remarkable success stories. You will read about one woman's incredible battle with breast and brain cancer and how she cured herself with coconut. This book includes an extensive A to Z reference with complete details on how to use coconut to prevent and treat dozens of common health problems.

Statements made in this book are documented with references to hundreds of published medical studies. The foreword is written by Dr. Conrado Dayrit, the first person to publish studies showing the benefit of coconut oil in treating HIV patients.

"As a doctor I have found coconut oil to be very useful. It has been of great help in treating hypertension, high cholesterol, and thyroid dysfunction as well as many other conditions. I highly recommend that you read this book."
Edna Aricaya-Huevos, MD

"Coconut oil has an important medical role to play in nutrition, metabolism, and health care. Indeed, properly formulated and utilized,

165

coconut oil may be the preferred vegetable oil in our diet and the special hospital foods used promoting patient recovery."
Conrado S. Dayrit, MD

"Excellent book. It is very helpful for those seeking to improve their health using natural medicine. I am actively conducting clinical trials and medical research using coconut oil and have seen very positive results with my patients."
Marieta Jader-Onate, MD

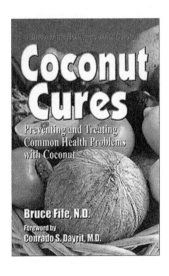

Coconut Cures is available from the publisher at www. piccadillybooks.com or from Amazon at https://goo.gl/WfvW4Y.

VIRGIN COCONUT OIL
Nature's Miracle Medicine
By Bruce Fife, ND

For countless generations virgin coconut oil has been used throughout the world as a nourishing food and a healing medicine. Its therapeutic use is described in ancient medical texts from India, Egypt, and China. Among the Pacific Islanders coconut is regarded as a sacred food. The oil is highly revered for its healing properties and forms the basis for nearly all of their traditional cures and therapies.

Modern medical science is now unlocking the secrets to virgin coconut oil's miraculous healing powers. Coconut oil in one form or another is currently being used in medicines, baby formulas, sports and fitness products, hospital feeding formulas, and even as a weight loss aid. Many doctors and nutritionists consider it to be the healthiest of all oils.

This short 95-page introduction to the miracles of coconut oil is presented in a friendly, non-technical format for those who want the facts but don't want to wade through a lot of scientific explanations and medical facts. Instead, it is filled with fascinating success stories and incredible testimonials from real people in real life situations.

In this book you will discover how people are successfully using virgin coconut oil to prevent and treat high cholesterol, high blood pressure, arthritis, fibromyalgia, Candida, ulcers, herpes, allergies, psoriasis, influenza, diabetes, and much more.

This book makes an excellent companion to *The Coconut Oil Miracle* or *Coconut Cures*. Contains different information.

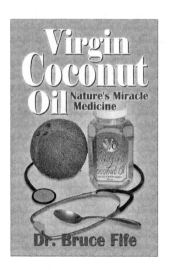

Virgin Coconut Oil is available from the publisher at www. piccadillybooks.com or from Amazon at https://goo.gl/uK1NTv.

References

Chapter 2: The Miracle of Fasting

1. Stewart, WK and Fleming, LW. Features of a successful therapeutic fast of 382 days' duration. *Postgraduate Medical Journal* 1973;49:203-209.

2. Thomson, TJ, et al. Treatment of obesity by total fasting for up to 249 days. *Lancet* 1966;2:992-996.

3. Garnett, ES, et al. Gross fragmentation of cardiac myofibrils after therapeutic starvation for obesity. *Lancet* 1969;1:914-916.

4. Runcie, J and Thomson, TJ. Prolonged starvation—a dangerous procedure? *British Medical Journal* 1970;3;432-435.

5. Lawler, DF, et al. Diet restriction and ageing in the dog: major observations over two decades. *B J Nutr* 2008;99:793-805.

6. Kjeldsen-Kragh, J, et al. Changes in laboratory variables in rheumatoid arthritis patients during a trial of fasting and one-year vegetarian diet. *Scand J Rheumatol* 1995;24:85-93.

7. Muller, H, et al. Fasting followed by vegetarian diet in patients with rheumatoid arthritis: a systematic review. *Scand J Rheumatoid* 2001;30:1-10.

8. Goldhammer, AC, et al. Medically supervised water-only fasting in the treatment of borderline hypertension. *J Altern Complement Med* 2002;8:643-650.

9. Masuda, A, et al. Cognitive behavioral therapy and fasting therapy for a patient with chronic fatigue syndrome. *Intern Med (Tokyo, Japan)* 2001:40;1158-1161.

10. Beer, AM, et al. Progression of intestinal secretory immunoglobulin A and the condition of the patients during naturopathic therapy and fasting therapy. *Forsch Komplementarmed Klass Naturheilkd* 2001;8:346-353.

11. Yamamoto, H., et al. Psychophysiological study on fasting therapy. *Psychother Psychosom* 1979;32:1-4.

12. Intermountain Medical Center. Routine periodic fasting is good for your health, and your heart, study suggests. *ScienceDaily*, 20 May 2011. www.sciencedaily.com/releases/2011/04/110403090259.htm.

13. Walford, RL. Calorie restriction: eat less, eat better, live longer. *Life Extension* 1998;Feb:19-22.

14. Bruce-Keller, AJ, et al. Food restriction reduces brain damage and improves behavioral outcome following excitotoxic and metabolic insults. *Ann Neurol* 1999;45:8-15.

15. Dubey, A, et al. Effect of age and caloric intake on protein oxidation in different brain regions and on behavioral functions of the mouse. *Arch Biochem Biophys* 1996;333:189-197.

Chapter 3: The Ketogenic Diet

1. Cahill, G.F. Jr. and Veech, R.L. Ketoacids? Good medicine? *Trans Am Clin Climatol Assoc* 2003;114:149-161.

2. Whitmer, R.A. Type 2 diabetes and risk of cognitive impairment and dementia. *Curr Neurol Neurosci Rep* 2007;7:3730380.

3. Ott, A, et al. Diabetes and the risk of dementia: Rotterdam study. *Neurology* 1999;53:1937-1942.

4. Xu, W, et al. Mid- and late-life diabetes in relation to the risk of dementia: a population-based twin study. *Diabetes* 2009;58:71-77.

5. de la Monte, SM, et al. Impaired insulin and insulin-like growth factor expression and signaling mechanisms in Alzheimer's disease—is this type 3 diabetes? *J Alzheimers Dis* 2005;7:63-80.

6. Sandyk, R. The relationship between diabetes mellitus and Parkinson's disease. *Int. J Neurosci* 1993;69:125-130.

7. Reyes, ET, et al. Insulin resistance in amyotrophic lateral sclerosis. *J Neurol Sci* 1984;63:317-324.

8. Hubbard, RW, et al. Elevated plasma glucagon in amyotrophic lateral sclerosis. *Neurology* 1992;42:1532-1534.

9. Kossoff, EH, et al. Ketogenic diets: an update for child neurologists. *J Child Neurol* 2009;24:979-88.

Chapter 4: Traditional Diets

1. Poti, JM, et al. Ultra-processed food intake and obesity: what really matters for health-processing or Nutrient content? *Curr Obes Rep* 2017;6:420-431.

2. Kim, H, et al. Ultra-processed food intake and mortality in the USA: results from the Third National Health and Nutrition Examination Survery (NHANES lll, 1988-1994). *Public Health Nutr* 2019; doi: 10.1017/S1368980018003890.

3. Schnabel, L, et al. Association between ultraprocessed food consumption and risk of mortality among middle-aged adults in France. *JAMA Intern Med* doi:10.1001/jamainternmed.2018.7289.

4. Pamplona, R, et al. Low fatty acid unsaturation: a mechanism for lowered lipoperoxidative modification of tissue proteins in mammalian species with long life spans. *J Gerontol A Biol Sci Med Sci* 2000;55:B286-B291.

5. Cha, YS and Sachan, DS. Opposite effects of dietary saturated and unsaturated fatty acids on ethanol-pharmacokinetics, triglycerides and carnitines. *J Am Coll Nutr* 1994;13:338-343.

6. Siri-Tarino, PW, et al. Meta-analysis of prospective cohort studies evaluating the association of saturated fat with cardiovascular disease. *American Journal of Clinical Nutrition* 2010;91:535-546.

7. Chowdhury, R, et al. Association of dietary, circulating, and supplement fatty acids with coronary risk: a systematic review and meta-analysis. *Ann Intern Med* 2014;160:398-406.

8. Grasgruber, P, et al. Good consumption and the actual statistics of cardiovascular diseases: an epidemiological comparison of 42 European countries. *Food Nutr Res* 2016 Sep 27;60:31694. Doi: 10.3402/fnr.v60.31694.

9. Ramsden, CE, et al. Use of dietary linoleic acid for secondary prevention of coronary heart disease and death: evaluation of recovered data from the Sydney Diet Heart Study and updated meta-analysis. *BMJ* 2013 Feb 4;346:e8707. Doi: 10.1136/bmj.e8707.

Chapter 5: Keto Cycling

1. Fife, B. *Ketone Therapy: The ketogenic Cleanse and Anti-Aging Diet.* Piccadilly Books, Ltd: Colorado Springs, CO 2017.

2. Muraro, PA, et al. *JAMA Neurol* 2017 Feb 20. doi: 10.1001/jamaneurol.2016.5867.

3. Cheng, CW, et al. Fasting-mimicking diet promotes Ngn3-driven beta-cell regeneration to reverse diabetes. *Cell* 2017;168:775-788.

4. Rangan, P, et al. Fasting-mimicking diet modulates microbiota and promotes intestinal regeneration to reduce inflammatory bowel disease pathology. *Cell Rep* 2019;26:2704-2719.

Chapter 6: The Healing Process

1.Magalle, L, et al. Intense sweetness surpasses cocaine reward. *PLoS One* 2007;8:e698.

2. https://www.gmwatch.org/en/news/latest-news/17932-exposure-prevalence-to-glyphosate-has-increased-500-since-introduction-of-gm-crops.

3. http://articles.latimes.com/2005/jul/22/nation/na-chemicals22.

4. https://www.nationalgeographic.com/science/health-and-human-body/human-body/chemicals-within-us/

5. Fife, B. *Ketone Therapy: The Ketogenic Cleanse and Anti-Aging Diet*. Piccadilly Books, Ltd.: Colorado Springs, CO; 2017.

6. Kashiwaya, Y, et al. D-beta-hydroxybutyrate protects neurons in models of Alzheimer's and Parkinson's disease. *Proc Natl Acad Sci USA* 2000;97:5440-5444.

7. Anson, RM, et al. Intermittent fasting dissociates beneficial effects of dietary restriction on glucose metabolism and neuronal resistance to injury from calorie intake. *Proc Natl Acad Sci USA* 2003;100:6216-6220.

8. Singh Baiwa, SJ, et al. Management of celphos poisoning with a novel intervention: a ray of hope in the darkest of clouds. *Anesth Essays Res* 2010;4:20-24.

Chapter 7: Low-Calorie Sweeteners: Friend or Foe?

1. http://stroke.ahajournals.org/content/early/2017/04/20/STROKEAHA.116.016027.

2. Fowler, SP, et al. Fueling the obesity epidemic? Artificially sweetened beverage use and long-term weight gain. *Obesity (Silver Spring, MD)* 2008;16:1894-1900.

3. Forshee, RA and Storey, ML. Total beverage consumption and beverage choices among children and adolescents. *Int J Food Sci Nutr* 2003;54:297–307.

4. Zarychanski, R, et al. Nonnutritive sweeteners and cardiometabolic health: a systematic review and meta-analysis of randomized controlled trials and prospective cohort studies. *CMAJ* 2017;189:E929-939.

5. Gardner, C, et al. American Heart Association Nutrition Committee of the Council on Nutrition, Physical Activity and Metabolism, Council on Arteriosclerosis, Thrombosis and Vascular Biology, Council on Cardiovascular Disease in the Young; American Diabetes Association. Nonnutritive sweeteners: current use and health perspectives: a scientific statement from the American Heart Association and the American Diabetes Association. *Diabetes Care* 2012;35(8):1798-1808.

6. Swithers SE. Artificial sweeteners produce the counterintuitive effect of inducing metabolic derangements. *Trends Endocrinol Metab* 2013;24:431-41.

7. Nettleton, JE, et al. Reshaping the gut microbiota: Impact of low calorie sweeteners and the link to insulin resistance? *Physiol Behav* 2016; 164(Pt B):488-93.

8. Fowler, SP. Low-calorie sweetener use and energy balance: results from experimental studies in animals, and large-scale prospective studies in humans. *Physiol Behav* 2016;164(Pt B):517-23.

9. Wang, Qiao-Ping, et al. Sucralose promotes food intake through NPY and a neuronal fasting response. *Cell Metabolism* 2016;24:75-90.

10. Bleich, SN, et al. Diet-beverage consumption and caloric intake among US adults, overall and by body weight. *Am J Public Health* 2014;104(3):e72-8.

11. Fife, B. *The Stevia Deception: The Hidden Dangers of Low-Calorie Sweeteners*. Piccadilly Books, Ltd.: Colorado Springs, CO., 2017.

12. Proceedings of the European Association for the Study of Diabetes, Lisbon, Portugal, September 13, 2017.

13. Suez, J, et al. Artificial sweeteners induce glucose intolerance by altering the gut microbiota. *Nature* 2014;514:181-186.

14. Azad, Meghan B, et al. Association between artificially sweetened beverage consumption during pregnancy and infant body mass index. *JAMA Pediatrics* 2016;170:662-670.

15. Fife, B. *The Stevia Deception: The Hidden Dangers of Low-Calorie Sweeteners*. Piccadilly Books, Ltd; Colorado Springs, CO; 2017.

16. Kimata, H. Anaphylaxis by stevioside in infants with atopic eczema. *Allergy* 2007;62:565-572.

17. Chan, P, et al. A double-blind placebo-controlled study of the effectiveness and tolerability of oral stevioside in human hypertension. *Br J Clin Pharmacol* 2000;50:215-220.

Chapter 8: Keto Mistakes

1. Dell, CA, et al. Lipid and fatty acid profiles in rats consuming different high-fat ketogenic diets. *Lipids* 2001;36:373-374.

2. Reger, MA, et al. Effects of beta-hydroxybutyrate on cognition in memory-impaired adults. *Neurobiol Aging* 2004;25:311-314.

3. Likhodii, SS, et al. Dietary fat, ketosis, and seizure resistance in rats on the ketogenic diet. *Epilepsia* 2000;41:1400-1410.

4. Taboulet, P. et al. Correlation between urine ketones (acetoacetate) and capillary blood ketones (3-beta-hydroxybutyrate) in hyperglycaemic patients. *Diabetes Metab* 2007;33:135-139.

5. Fife, B. *The Coconut Ketogenic Diet: Supercharge Your Metabolism, Revitalize Thyroid Function, and Lose Excess Weight.* Piccadilly Books, Ltd.: Colorado Springs, CO; 2014.

6. Roberts, MN, et al. A ketogenic diet extends longevity and healthspan in adult mice. *Cell Metab* 2017;26:539-546.

Index

A1C, 6
Acetoacetate, 28, 128
Acetone, 28
Alpha-linolenic acid, 56
Alzheimer's disease, 33
Amyloid plaque, 22
Ancestral diets, 47-48, 63
Antioxidants, 60, 70, 96
Atkins, Robert, 37, 110
Autoimmune disorders, 72
Autophagy, 22, 66, 69-75

Bad breath, 90
Barbieri, Angus, 12-13
Belly fat, 10
Beta-hydroxybutyrate, 28, 126, 128, 140
Brain derived neurotrophic factors, 28, 96
Brain health, 33-34
Brain natriuretic peptide (BNP), 116

Calorie restriction, 18-21, 23
Capric acid, 57
Caprylic acid, 57
Carbohydrate, 29-30, 118-119
Carotenoids, 60
Catalase, 96
Chemotherapy, 71-72
Cholesterol, 61, 119-120
Christopher, John R., 80
Classic ketogenic diet, 26-29, 35
Coconut ketogenic diet, 38

Coconut oil, 36-37, 38, 58, 125, 135
Conditionally essential fatty acids, 57-58
Constipation, 89, 138
Cooklin, Hugh, 26

Degenerative disease, 43
Detoxification, 94-100
Diabetes, 6-8, 17, 32-33, 73-74, 106
Diabetic neuropathy, 33
Diarrhea, 136
Digestive function, 89
Disease crisis, 97-98
Diseases of modern civilization, 43
Dr. Atkins' New Diet Revolution, 37, 110
Duncan, David, 91-92

Electrolytes, 41, 89, 136
Epilepsy, 26-27, 29, 37-38
Essential fatty acids, 56
Exogenous ketones, 139-141

Fasting, 12-25, 27, 69-75
Fasting blood glucose, 32
Fasting Cure, The, 16
Fasting mimicking diet, 74-76, 84, 142-148
Fat, 29-30, 52-62, 136
Fatty acids, 53
Fiber, 39, 132

Fractionated coconut oil, 36
Freeman, John, 110
Free radicals, 54, 70
Fructose, 30
Fruit, 40

Galactose, 30
Geylin, H. Rawle, 26
Glucagon, 31
Gluconeogenesis, 69
Glucosis, 5, 27, 30, 77
Glutathione, 96
Glycogen, 30
Glyphosate, 91
Gut microbiome, 75, 110, 113, 137-138

Healing crisis, 96-100
Heart disease, 8, 17, 61-62, 67, 115-116
HDL cholesterol, 120
Human growth hormone (HGH), 17-18
Huttenlocher, Peter, 36
Hydrogenated vegetable oil, 54-55
Hypothyroidism 133-135

Inflammatory bowel disease (IBD), 75
Insulin, 30-32
Insomnia, 89
Insulin resistance, 32-35
Intermittent fasting, 6, 23-25, 64
Inuit, 120

Ketoacidosis, 127-128
Keto breath, 90

Keto cycling, 5-11, 63-86, 123
Keto flu, 90, 96
Ketogenic Diet: A Treatment for Epilepsy, The, 110
Keto junk foods, 109, 130-131
Ketone bodies, 28
Ketones, 5, 28, 37, 76, 70-71, 87-90, 94-96, 119, 127-129
Ketone esters, 140
Ketone salts, 140
Ketosis test strips, 42, 128--129

Lactose, 30
Lauric acid, 57
LDL cholesterol, 120
linoleic acid, 56
Long chain fatty acids, 36, 53
Longo, Valter, 70-76, 95
Low-fat diets, 60

Macfadden, Bernarr, 15-16
Magnesium, 41, 136, 138
Malnutrition, 19, 50-51
McCay, C.M., 18
MCT ketogenic diet, 35-37
MCT oil, 36-37
Medium chain fatty acids, 53, 57-58
Medium chain triglycerides (MCTs), 35-37
Modified Atkins diet, 37-38
Monk fruit extract, 111
Monounsaturated fatty acids, 53-54, 59, 124
Multiple sclerosis (MS), 72-73
Muscle cramps, 89

Net carbohydrate, 39

Nonnutritive sweeteners, 103-117
Nutrition and Physical Degeneration, 47
Nutritional ketosis, 5, 37, *see also* ketosis

Obesity, 17, 34-35, 105, 106-107

Paleo diet, 47
Palm kernel oil, 58
Peterman, Mynie, 29
Phthalates, 92
Physical culture, 15-16
Polybrominated diphenyl ethers, 93
Polyunsaturated fatty acids, 53-54, 59
Potassium, 41, 136
Price, Weston A., 44-46
Processed meats, 40
Prostate, 112-114
Protein, 29-30, 40, 119, 123
PSA, 113-114

Rebaudioside A, 112
Roundup, 91

Salt, 41, 136
Saturated fats, 61-62, 119-120, *see also* saturated fatty acids
Saturated fatty acids, 53-54, 58, 59, 124, *see also* saturated fats
Short chain fatty acids, 53
Sinclair, Upton, 16
Sodium, 41, 136
Sorbitol, 110

Starch, 30, 50
Stem cells, 64-69, 75
Stevia, 110-117
Steviol glycosides, 112
Stevioside, 112
Subclinical malnutrition, 51, 133
Sugar, 30, 62, 88, 101-102
Sugar addiction, 88, *see also* sweet addiction
Sugar alcohols, 102
Sugar metabolism, 29-30
Sugar substitutes, 102-103, 129-130
Superoxide dismutase, 96
Sweet addiction, 107-109

Therapeutic fasting 14-18, 26-27
Thirst, 89
Thyroid, 133-135
Toxins, 90-96
Traditional fats, 52-53
Trans fatty acids, 54
Triglyceride, 56

Ultra-processed foods, 48-52
Urine test strips, 42

Vegetable oils, 53-54, 59, 123-124, 134
Vertigo, 115
Visceral fat, 10

Walford, Roy L., 20
Weight loss, 121-122
Weston A. Price Foundation, 48
Wilder, Russel, 29

Xylitol, 110

Printed in Great Britain
by Amazon

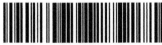